The Happy, H. Mom

Recovery, well-being and weight loss after childbirth

By

Miriam McKnight

The Healthy, Happy, Mom

Recovery, well-being and weight loss after childbirth

Miriam McKnight

The Healthy, Happy, Mom
Recovery, well-being and weight loss after
childbirth
By Miriam McKnight
Cover design by margethechicken

Disclaimer

No part of this publication or the information in it may be quoted from or reproduced in any form by means such as printing, scanning, photocopying or otherwise without prior written permission of the copyright holder.

Disclaimer and Terms of Use: Effort has been made to ensure that the information in this book is accurate and complete, however, the author and the publisher do not warrant the accuracy of the information, text and graphics contained within the book due to the rapidly changing nature of science, research, known and unknown facts, and the internet. The Author and the publisher do not hold any responsibility for errors, omissions or contrary interpretation of the subject matter herein. This book is presented solely for motivational and informational purposes only.

And just to let you know, there are no sales pitches and no affiliate links within this book. All the information is here to help you and not for me to sell more products!

TABLE OF CONTENTS

My values

I do not believe in perfection. No one is perfect. I do not believe your appearance dictates your value. You are already wonderfully precious. I want you to run away from comparison. Comparison is crippling and besides, the woman you perceive as Beautiful Super Mom, probably feels far from super. Happiness is not dependent on looking good, nor do I think that skinny is best.

You are brilliant! You are lovely! You are an amazing mom!

Whoever you are, whether rich or poor, athletic or overweight, chilled or stressed, happy or unhappy, I have written this book to encourage you to value who you are and value your health. Through valuing yourself in this way you will honor your family too. It is my desire that you recover well, regain fitness and feel happy during your first years as a mom! A happy, healthy, mom is best for everyone!

Having had 3 boys I understand the constant demands and never ending labors of love as a mom. All too often we find that our needs and desires are put on hold. However, when it comes down to health, fitness and happiness I simply know that you need to intentionally make time and space for yourself. You are important and you are worth it. I want to help you love yourself and love your life!

I know moms do not have much time to themselves so I have done the work for you. I have taken the time to find out what exactly works best for moms. How to recover well from birth, how to look after your changed hair and skin, and how to regain fitness and get that amazing body back. I have explored the common struggles and challenges that moms face and how best to gain a healthy lifestyle that works for you and your family.

Be healthy and happy, look good and feel great! Xxx

Introduction

Welcome to The Healthy, Happy, Mom! I began thinking about writing this book after reflecting on my own experience as a mom, and having spoken to countless other moms who have struggled with the huge life change after having a baby. Feeling happy with yourself, your new life and your changed body can be a challenge! As a new mom, regaining your fitness, losing weight and getting back in to shape seems like a selfish focus, yet I believe prioritizing yourself during this time reaps multitudes of benefits. I have so much respect and admiration for moms whom selflessly give of themselves day after day. I want to help those who continuously spend their time serving, helping and loving others. Because moms have so little time to invest in themselves, I want to offer quality, precise information and advice that will have a direct impact on recovery, well-being and weight loss after childbirth. My desire to cover relevant topics that impact well-being will help prepare you for the changes and challenges that will arise. I want to provide something that is clear, simple to understand and easy to follow. I can give you mountains of motivation and of course results! I believe that getting back into shape after having your baby will improve your overall quality of life. Not only is it about what you look like, but about boosting your health and happiness too!

I am going to share my experiences, things I've

learned, read, researched and tried over the course of having 3 boys. I want to encourage you and say that you can reach your goal. By following these simple guidelines and advice, you will be able to be the happy yummy mommy that you've always wanted to be. I even believe that with a few easy steps you can look even better than you did before you were pregnant! Throughout my whole life, although not some crazy fitness dude, I have loved sport and being active. Personally, deciding to have children felt like a huge sacrifice. I believed I would never again have the pre-pregnancy body that I had. I thought pregnancy was the end of enjoying an athletic slim physique. I simply didn't realize it didn't have to be that way! I am actually more body content now than ever before! Take heart!

Your body has been through a tough nine months. Yes, it has been an incredible awe-inspiring experience (especially seeing the outcome), but it has been hard work too. Your body has coped with the changing hormones, which has affected how you look and feel. It has carried the extra weight, which has put extra pressure on your back and hips. Pregnancy has affected your skin and hair too. Your nutrient reserves are low. Even your lungs have worked extra hard – I frequently complained I could not keep up with the apparently slow walking pace my husband was setting. Simply bending to pick something off the floor was a massive task! Yes, carrying a baby is a natural process, but one that has left our bodies with much healing, recovery and redefining to be done!

It seems unfair. Your body has worked hard to make a baby, and then you have to work hard again to get it back to how you want it. Unfortunately it's not going to happen automatically, though I wish it did. You simply have to put the work in. I wrote this guide to enable you to return your body to as close to its pre-pregnancy state as possible. But don't be mistaken that pre-pregnancy is always better. Many women who have followed these guidelines have ended up with **better** bodies after having children than before. It's an opportunity for a change. Take it!

Never think about waiting to get back in to shape after having all the kids you want ... huge error! It will be so much harder to get your body back after multiple pregnancies. In addition to the bad habits you will form, and the extra weight you will gain, you will be older in years and thus it is harder to boost your metabolism, lose weight and see skin rejuvenated! In fact my advice is think about your post-pregnancy body before you even get pregnant! Get in to the shape of your life before you conceive. This will help in numerous ways. Firstly you will see how amazing you can look, which will really inspire you to regain it! Secondly you will have established good exercise and eating habits that will continue into your pregnancy. Thirdly, because you have started with good muscle tone, your body will have a good metabolic rate throughout pregnancy, helping less fat to be stored. Good core muscle tone will also help to avoid suffering back pain. Fourthly, by starting with no extra weight, you will ultimately be less stretched at the end of your pregnancy, leaving less weight to lose after birth to regain your shape. Furthermore, the less stretched your skin has been the more likely it will make a good recovery. Bonus!

Once the baby is born it takes a bit of time to get into a routine before you can start implementing the advice and actions in this book. The key is patience, perseverance, and prioritize! Bit by bit you can do it! The Social Readjustment Rating Scale (SRRS) popularly known as the Holmes and Rahe Stress Scale is a list of 43 stressful life events that can contribute to illness. Pregnancy comes in at number 12, and the addition of a new member to the family at number 14, both pretty high up the scale! These events, along with the knock-on life changes that come from having a baby, can all add up and accumulate in a number of "Life Change Units", which have shown to be correlated with developing stress related illnesses. Therefore it is vital to take care of yourself and to slowly adjust to this new way of life, making sure your health and well-being is prioritized. Often becoming a new mom requires us to bring more routine into our daily life. Children often like to eat and sleep at similar times each day. I am naturally a spontaneous person, not liking to over plan my life, but we can and should use routine to our benefit. It may allow us to plan in regular times to exercise, cook the right food, or get some "me" time. All of these are important factors that contribute to our overall well-being.

My motivation for writing this book is to help moms feel good about themselves, and to live a happy and fulfilled life. There are enough stressful things in life without having to worry about health, weight and appearance. I am only too aware that it is pretty tough for moms. There's so much to adjust to. It's so hard balancing it all; looking after the children, family admin, finances, household chores, going back to work, school runs, shopping, getting up in the night, cooking, cleaning, and washing ... It's important to know you're not alone. Millions of moms struggle with the same demands and stresses, leaving little time and energy to focus on their own health and happiness. Many moms want to regain their fitness and figure and when they do have a moment to think about this, they don't know where to start. Therefore I've done the work so you don't have to. I've found out what works and what doesn't, so all you have to do is read the information, and apply it to your life. It's my genuine desire to see moms looking great, enjoying life, loving their kids and families, and not struggling with their health and well-being. Why should we have to lug around excess weight, suffer with bad skin, feel constantly tired, have an ever-slowing metabolism, be run-down by work or home life, and not look good? I want you to be proud of your family and yourself. I want you to be so happy and full of life and energy that you are able to give help and advice to others who are struggling. I want you to recognize the value that you bring to this world and know that you are special and certainly deserve time and attention too.

Lots of books give plenty general advice and encouragement, but leave you with plenty of questions in your head about the specifics. In this book, I will give you general advice and guidelines, AND concrete steps to follow.

This book will give results! Have fun!

Miri xx

Chapter 1 - Rest, Recovery and Sleep!

It is a well-known fact that women need lots of rest and sleep in the days immediately following the birth of a child. It is important for the healing of your body, production of milk, and for your general day-to-day functioning. It also has a direct impact on your eventual ability to lose weight and get in to shape. Not everyone realizes that it's not only important immediately after the birth, but continues to be a valuable aspect of your general health and well-being months after too. Let's look at some of the specific details of healing, rest and sleep to help us understand the significance of this.

Rest and recovery

My intention is not to give you medical advice here. I do however, want to make you aware of the natural processes your body is going through, preparing you for what is to come and how you may be able to best cope with this new phase in your life.

During pregnancy your uterus has grown about 1000 times larger than usual. Right after childbirth the uterus can be felt level with the belly button, but immediately following this it begins to contract, causing the uterus to expel the placenta. Women can often receive an injection of Syntometrine to help the placenta come out quickly. At this point, the uterus feels like a hard mass in the middle of the abdomen. After the placenta is expelled, a process called *involution* begins, where it shrinks down to its original size and eventually fits back underneath the pubic bone. This process starts immediately but it takes about 8 weeks for a woman's uterus to regain its pre-pregnancy size.

The contractions that cause involution can be quite uncomfortable and even painful. Some women say that these contractions feel like menstrual cramps, while others would describe them as being similar to the contractions of childbirth! These after pains may be felt more intensely following second and subsequent births. In my experience these cramps were agony! After I gave birth to my third son, Titus, I remember asking the nurse if I could continue using the gas and air to manage the pain! At home, even days later, breastfeeding would trigger these painful cramps. I may not be the toughest person in the world, but it did really hurt and felt like labor all over again. As I lay there doubled over in pain, sweating and moaning I tried to focus on the fact that if my uterus was shrinking, then so was my belly!

For the first few days of being a mom, the breasts tend to be soft but a little tender. The body is producing colostrum, a thin, clear-yellow liquid that is high in protein. This precedes the more mature milk in breastfeeding moms. At around day three or four your breasts begin to produce milk. Your breasts grow big, full and firm! A brilliant look, but pretty painful I'm afraid! Yet it is a matter of days before this hardness and discomfort will subside. In the meantime it may help to express a little before latching your baby on to feed.

Following labor, most women feel exhausted and continue to feel some discomfort depending on the type of birth they experienced. I do not intend to instill any fear in you, but I do want to be honest. Even following the most straightforward 'easy' births, women tend to feel bruised, swollen and delicate. In the more difficult and complicated births women can be left feeling really damaged. Physically and emotionally they feel much pain. Having a caesarean, an episiotomy or experiencing a first, second or third degree tear is more than uncomfortable for a good while. When I gave birth to Jonah I was given an episiotomy and was therefore given stitches. I was stitched neatly but unfortunately too tightly. I felt continuously uncomfortable for fourteen months until I gave birth to my second son, Levi. I know others who have struggled with their stitches becoming infected, others coping with catheters, constipation or swollen legs. Some suffer from mastitis, where your breasts can become painful and you can experience a high temperature and feel ill. All women will have vaginal discharge called lochia, which is the tissue and blood that lined your uterus during pregnancy. It is heavy and bright red at first, becoming lighter in flow and color until it comes to an end a few weeks later. My point being, birth is not easy. Dealing with pain is exhausting and recovery takes time. You are also coping with the added responsibility of caring for a newborn and all the life changes that come along with it!

Different cultures round the world have different traditions and beliefs about the initial period following the birth of a child. A brief look at some of them gives an interesting insight into the topic and a comparison of practices.

- In China, women generally rest for 30 days after giving birth. The housework is taken care of by female relatives or live-in helpers.

- Midwives in Guatemala, traditionally visit new moms every day for the first 2 to 3 weeks. They check the health of the mom and baby AND give the mom a massage AND take care of all the housework enabling the mother to rest.

- In India and much of South East Asia, the mother and baby are secluded for up to 40 days. This post partum confinement is believed to protect the mother and baby from exposure to illnesses as well as evil spirits at this time when both are in a vulnerable state. If they are not leaving the house, I gather they are not pushing themselves too hard and are getting plenty of rest!

- In many countries in the Middle East, it is customary to rest for 40 days after the birth.

The housework, care of other children, and taking care of the new baby is done by a friend or member of the family who comes and stays at the house during this period.

- In Mayan Indian culture in Mexico, the mother only resumes normal activities after the baby is 20 days old. For them, this marks the end of the pregnancy and childbirth process, which culminates in the mother receiving a massage from the midwife. During the first 7 days of this time, the mother and new baby remain indoors and contact with visitors is kept to a minimum.

In contrast, women in the West are often expected to put on a brave face and just get on with it. We tend to resume normal activities almost immediately. Looking after the baby and our older children, housework, shopping, cooking, driving. ... We do have visits from midwives and health care professionals, but these visits are contained to health checks and some emotional support. While this resumption of daily life may be possible, is it really necessary? Shouldn't we take longer to make sure that we get adequate rest and heal properly? If possible, I would encourage you to get as much help as you can over these first few days and weeks. Don't wait until you have pushed yourself to the edge and feel completely overwhelmed and exhausted.

The combination of changing hormone levels and the physical and emotional demands on a new mom can lead to 'baby blues'. This is experienced by 8 out of 10 moms and resting helps get over this. If the 'baby blues' persist it can lead to postnatal depression. If you have severe feelings of depression, guilt, and sadness or you feel you just cannot cope; you simply must seek help from your health professional. Some women don't talk about such feelings as they feel ashamed and embarrassed that they feel this way. Don't let this happen to you. You haven't done anything wrong. Just get help. Postnatal depression can make it hard to care for your baby and establish a close bond. Your feelings of self worth and happiness are key to achieving good post pregnancy health too. Ensure you get support and advice to help you get through this. Give yourself the space and time to not only relax physically but mentally and emotionally too. When you are well rested your body heals better, milk production is better, you will regain energy and strength, you will feel more able to cope and you will be a better mom, partner and friend!

Sleep

Studies show that anything less than 6 hours of sleep per night can be hazardous to a person's health and safety. It is easy to see that a massive change to our life as a parent is adapting to both a new sleep pattern and lack of sleep! There will be times when you can't remember what serenity felt like. You soon learn that a baby has a different body clock to us. Typically a newborn will awaken every 2-3 hours and needs changing, feeding, maybe changing again, comforting and so on. This routine doesn't confine itself to daytime hours either, but continues 24hours a day (almost certainly for the first few weeks at least). Be under no illusion, even the best sleeping babies will still have some level of impact on your sleep, and the more unsettled sleepers will have a huge impact! Alas, the amount of sleep a person needs increases if they have been deprived during the previous days. So basically you create a 'sleep debt' that builds up and eventually needs to be repaid. You cannot truly adapt to getting too little sleep. It may seem like you adapt, by getting used to the sleep deprived schedule, but you will remain affected by it.

A few months after my first son was born I remember after one night time feed I refilled my pint glass with water, and in a confused state walked over to the toilet and dropped it down the bowl making such a loud smashing noise that my husband darted through in a complete panic. I did not flinch. I did not move a muscle. I didn't even curse. I was so tired my body nor brain couldn't respond in any way whatsoever. I believe most new moms could tell numerous stories of moments of complete tiredness when things go a little pear shaped! It's not unusual. In fact it is totally normal. You are probably already aware of the side effects of too little sleep. None are pleasant and some are more serious than others.

Side effects of too little sleep

Fine and gross motor impairment (beware, this can affect your ability to drive safely!)

Clumsiness

Slowed reaction time

Overreactions

Hallucinations

Paranoia

Increase in tension

Headaches

Memory problems

Fatigue

Inability to concentrate

High blood pressure

Low sex drive

Depression

Feeling grumpy, groggy, impatient, irritable, and moody

Impairment of judgment and interpretation of

events. (Sleep deprived people are particularly poor at assessing what the lack of sleep is doing to them. Therefore you may not be aware that you need help).

A weakening of your immune system, increasing your chance of becoming ill

Increase in perception of pain

Daytime sleepiness

Weight gain – Recent research has looked at the link between sleep and appetite. Shortened periods of sleep are associated with an increase in appetite and increase in cravings for high-fat, high-carbohydrate foods. Interestingly, research studies are even considering whether adequate sleep should be prescribed as a standard part of weight loss programs!

Wrinkles- yes, I said wrinkles! It is during deep sleep that growth hormone is released. This is needed for normal tissue repair. Without it, the skin begins to age, developing lines, which become wrinkles. The stress hormone cortisol, released when you are sleep deprived can break down skin collagen, the protein that keeps skin smooth and elastic!

Additionally, chronic sleep deprivation has been shown to increase risk factors for obesity, diabetes, heart disease, cancer and accidents!

Having looked at the negative impact lack of

sleep has, let's take a look at the benefits of sleep and what is happening in the body during sleep. Whilst asleep, the body is under less demand and thus takes its opportunity to both rest and carry out functions that are difficult during waking hours.

Benefits of sleep

Energy stores in the muscles are replenished.

Damaged cells are destroyed whilst new cells are created.

Toxins are eliminated from your blood stream and muscles.

The brain reorganizes mental and emotional thoughts, which helps memory, learning and decision making when awake.

Needless to say, we should do all we can to help avoid being continuously sleep deprived. Having lived through the reality of having three babies in the space of four and a half years, I want to offer my help, advice and encouragement. At times it is tough, really tough. You need to respond to your baby's needs but at the same time protect yourself from becoming sleep deprived. We cannot wave a magic wand and expect a child to sleep 8 hours in a row every night, but we can do things to improve our situation and give us the best chance possible of getting the sleep required. I want to look at what you can change to allow for more sleep ... you are coping with a super busy schedule, but sleep should not be last on the agenda. Try some of the practical tips for the first few weeks

Practical Tips

Sleep when the baby sleeps. This may be only a few minutes rest several times a day, but these minutes can add up. Short bursts of sleep during the day are better than none at all. Get in to bed, close the curtains and make the environment as calming as possible so that you and your baby get good quality sleep.

Save time by being organized. Have your baby's bed near yours for feeding at night. My husband moved our newborn out of our room after the first night as he complained of waking every time the baby moved. So the deal was that he had to bring him to me to be fed in the night, and put him back after he was fed! If you too struggle with being easily awoken, consider moving the baby further away so you don't get disturbed every few minutes. Have a changing mat in a convenient place alongside everything else you need for changing. This will save precious minutes of sleep time at night!

When you can, introduce a bottle of expressed milk to breastfed babies for a night-time feed. This way, someone else can feed the baby, and you can have a longer period of uninterrupted sleep. For formula-fed babies, take advantage of others who are able to feed at night too.

Many new parents enjoy visits from friends and family, but don't exhaust yourself entertaining your guests. Feel free to excuse yourself for a nap whilst they tend to the baby. All parties will be happy!

Get outside for a few minutes each day. Fresh air and walking can make you feel refreshed and help you sleep better.

If you are breastfeeding, try using its calming effect to go to sleep straight after feeding, when your baby drops off to sleep.

Don't lie in bed watching TV or surfing the net thinking you are getting rest. Yes, it's more relaxing than rushing round the house doing chores but it's not sleep. Turn your devices off, turn the ringer off your phone, and go to sleep.

Early nights! Be disciplined. This is one thing that I was good at. I'm not a morning person, but my first and third children are, so I had to make sure I got to bed early to ensure that I could cope well the next day.

Take it in turns with your partner for "lie-ins". Utilize the weekends.

Don't be afraid to ask for help. Receiving home cooked meals from friends and family is most helpful! It really does free up time for sleep. Consider putting together a 7-day rota and asking your close friends and family to sign up to bring you an evening meal on one of these days during the first week of your new arrival.

Adapt your standards! If you are a person who loves an immaculate house, you may need to lower your standards temporarily! Do not put yourself under the pressure of doing everything you did before. OK, do what is essential in terms of cleaning and tidying but do not attempt any big tasks or a spring clean! These things can wait.

Organize your time. Make a list of everything you do, and want to spend time doing. Divide your list into essentials and non-essentials. Prioritize both lists. This means that when you have finished your essentials, you know which of the non-essentials you most want to do.

My essentials
(Yours can be different)

Caring for my new baby
Spending time with my other children and husband
Day-to-day house jobs like cooking and the essential cleaning
Food shopping
My sleep
"Me" time

When you have more routine, time and capacity you can fit in the non-essentials

Socializing / entertaining
Exercising
Hobbies
Personal projects
Work

Doing this should hopefully give you more time for sleep. You will find you have more time in the day as you will not be wasting time doing things that are not on your list. Knowing that you have been organized and have managed to do what you planned will help you have good quality sleep. You won't lie in bed feeling guilty thinking I should be doing this or that. You will feel you have deserved your sleep and be able to switch off. Considering you are now also more aware of the importance of sleep you should find it easier to prioritize it.

Much of this chapter has been dedicated to the first 6-8 weeks after childbirth. However the importance of rest and sleep remains throughout the rest of your life. Sleep is vital. Why am I so keen that you heal well and get plenty of sleep and rest? Because I want you to enjoy motherhood, love your baby, and get off to the good start you deserve. It will also allow you to apply the principles I am going introduce later, to get you well on your way to having the body you dreamed of! Rest and relaxation complement a fitness program. You must have both to rejuvenate your strength and vitality. Once you're well rested, you'll have the energy for a comprehensive exercise program. Look after your sleep and your beauty will begin to shine!

Chapter 2 - Breastfeeding

This book, including this chapter is primarily about you. Your health and your happiness, and not focused on your baby (when probably right now, a lot of things are). You are most likely already aware of the benefits of breastfeeding for your baby; general health, efficient digestion, reduced risk of allergies, good skin, strong immunity, higher IQ. ... But I want to focus on the best thing for YOU and when the benefits of having a healthy baby can have a positive impact on you.

It is now well documented that breastfeeding is as good for mothers as it is for babies. Lactation is said to be a continuation of the physiological processes started at conception, and it is a way of bringing closure to the process, and which allows the body to return to its pre-conception state. Some experts even call it the fourth trimester of pregnancy! Not breastfeeding after birth seems to put the mother at an increased risk of a number of serious diseases. The mechanisms behind these increased risks are still being researched, but experts think that by not engaging in the process that the body prepares for during pregnancy, many crucial systems can go out of synch. There are both long term and short-term benefits associated with breastfeeding. Let's take a look. ...

#1 Helps to prevent postpartum hemorrhaging

Mothers who breastfeed recover from childbirth more quickly and easily. Repeated suckling of the baby directly results in the mother's pituitary gland releasing the hormone oxytocin. Immediately after the birth of the baby, oxytocin plays an important role. Firstly, it signals to the breasts to release milk for the baby. Secondly, it simultaneously produces contractions to the uterus, which sends signals to the body to shut down blood supply to the vessels that nourished the growing baby, and thus preventing hemorrhaging. However, mothers who don't breastfeed can be given artificial oxytocin to avoid excessive hemorrhage.

#2 Uterus shrinks and returns back to normal

These contractions (as mentioned earlier) help prevent postpartum hemorrhaging and also help the uterus to contract and return to a non-pregnant size. This is a very important step in getting back to the shape you want! As your uterus gets smaller, so does your tummy! If a woman does not breastfeed, her uterus will remain slightly larger than it was before pregnancy.

#3 Return of menstrual period is delayed

When there is an absence of menstrual period (amenorrhea), it can help provide natural spacing of pregnancies. This healthy time gap between pregnancies is needed for a good physical recovery. Although this is a fairly reliable source of contraceptive, you can still get pregnant whilst breastfeeding (proved by myself)! So, if you do not want a baby soon, you should use back-up forms of contraceptive.

Throughout breastfeeding, the body conserves more iron than normal. We do lose some iron to breast milk, but this is not as much as the amount lost during normal periods. This decreases the risk of anemia. The longer the mother breastfeeds for, the stronger this effect. Your periods can return in six to eight weeks or sooner if you do not breastfeed. Your periods however, can return whilst still breastfeeding, but this usually occurs much later.

#4 Burns more calories

Breastfeeding causes you to burn up to 500 more calories per day. Yes, 500! The production of breast milk uses 200-500 calories per day, which would otherwise take a LOT of exercise to burn (approximately 45 minutes to an hour of exercise). Additionally, breastfeeding helps your metabolic profile, thus increasing fat loss. Quite simply breastfeeding is the best fat loss tool. In fact scientific studies show that non-breastfeeding moms lose less weight AND don't keep weight off as well as mothers whom breastfeed! I breastfed all three of my children and lost weight, regaining my pre-pregnancy weight on each occasion. This is what should happen for you. If you follow the guidelines in my chapter on eating and drinking, you should lose fat at a rate of about 1lb per week. Add in exercise at the right time and you will see fantastic results!

#5 Decreases risk of diabetes

Weight loss from breastfeeding can prevent mothers who have gestational diabetes from developing it later on in life. Studies show that these mothers have lower blood sugars than non-breastfeeding mothers.

Also, women with type 1 diabetes need less insulin when breastfeeding due to their reduced blood sugar levels.

#6 Reduces risk of heart attacks

The fact that breastfeeding produces the optimal level of weight loss, an improved control of blood sugar, and a good cholesterol profile could be contributing factors in reducing the risk of heart problems. This is particularly important, as heart attacks are a leading cause of death in women.

#7 Increase in bone density and reduced risk of osteoporosis

Despite the fact that calcium is needed in the production of breast milk, studies have revealed that after weaning, a mother's bone density returns to the same levels as before pregnancy, or even higher. Non-breastfeeding women have a four times greater chance of developing osteoporosis than breastfeeding women. Further studies have shown that women who did not breastfeed have a greater risk of hip fractures after menopause.

#8 Reduced risk of cancers

It has been estimated that breastfeeding for 6-24 months throughout your life can reduce the risks of breast cancer by 11-25%. Another study has shown that the risk of developing breast cancer can be reduced by almost 50% by breastfeeding. Whether it's 11 or 50%, any possible decrease in risk is worth knowing about! This decreased risk could be due to the reduced levels of estrogen during breastfeeding, and to the local effect of the natural physiological function of the breast.

Additionally, ovarian and uterine cancers have been found more common in non-breastfeeding mothers. Experts suggest this may be due to repeated ovulatory cycles and exposure to high levels of estrogen. Estrogen levels are lower during lactation, and this means there is less estrogen available to stimulate the lining of the uterus and perhaps breast tissue too, hence lessening the risk of these tissues becoming cancerous.

#9 Cost

If financial position may be a consideration for you, guess what.... breast milk is free! Whilst saving money on formula milk, you can spend it on good foods, vitamins, and supplements for yourself. Bear in mind, a baby who is less prone to need medical attention due to the health benefits breast milk gives, will in turn, save not just time and heartache, but also money.

#10 Convenience

Convenient is not a word I would use to describe life with a new baby. Gone are the days of grabbing your wallet, phone and car keys and heading out of the door! As a mom you now feel you have so much to think about and remember before you head out. Nappies, nappy bags, wet wipes, muslins, spare change of clothes (I was thinking for the baby, but I suppose some moms who might need to look super perfect may need to change if they get splattered with baby food or get a milky shoulder), dummy, snacks (for you and baby), blanket, toys ... the list goes on. I always felt privileged that bottles and formula for us were not on that list. It was just one less thing to have to remember, get ready and pack.

Psychological benefits

The purpose of this book is to deliver to you the best information on how to look good, and live a healthy, active life. Living a stress-free life, or more realistically, a less-stressed life, is one of the biggest factors in healthy living. Knowing that you are giving your baby the best possible start brings satisfaction and peace of mind. You are offering something that is natural, has the perfect ingredients, has the right blend, the right taste, and the right temperature. Breast milk not only gives baby optimal nutrition, and a protection from disease, but it creates opportunity to emotionally bond together. The intimacy of skin-to-skin contact and time with him/her creates a bond that is hard to replicate. This emotional connectedness creates feelings of joy, happiness, peace, fulfillment and contentment.

Both oxytocin and prolactin (the milk-making hormone), which are released when breastfeeding, have been shown to have calming and relaxing effects on mothers. They have even been found to lower blood pressure. This is invaluable during such demanding times of change. These hormones can also help establish a strong sense of love and attachment between you and your little one. Your time spent feeding is unique and special. No one else can spend time like that with your baby.

I don't intend to make you feel guilty if you are unable to breastfeed, or give you some kind of complex if you didn't choose to breastfeed. Maybe it wasn't for you. I know it is not best for everyone. Some moms find that choosing to formula feed their baby can lessen the pressure and stress of life with a newborn. It removes the pressure of being the only person that can feed the baby, which can bring increased feelings of freedom and peace of mind. For some moms, breastfeeding is physically too difficult or even impossible.

I do urge you not to give up on breastfeeding too soon. If you've tried it and its tough, take heart, as it does get better. It is certainly not easy when you first start! For the few, the baby takes to the nipple straight away and there are no problems. For many, it's not that simple. My son was unable to latch onto the nipple, and I had to use weird silicon nipple shields for the first few weeks. Practically, that made it awkward and tiresome. Having to locate the shields in the middle of the night when half asleep, sterilize them before every feed, balance them on my breast and then trying to latch him on, proved a pain in the butt. But in the end these shields proved to be a real help, and after a while my tiny baby boy was able to take to the nipple without help and he fed really well. I needed special cream for the soreness and cracks on my nipples but I am so pleased that I persevered and as a result I reaped all the benefits of breastfeeding. It would have been easier to have given up and have given him a bottle. But I really wanted to breastfeed him and so that's what I did. So please persevere with it. It may be difficult and even feel unnatural to start with, but keep trying and you won't regret it.

Consider breastfeeding. Your baby will be healthier and happier, and so will you!

Chapter 3 - "Me" Time!

The early months of being a new mom, although exhilarating, pleasurable and satisfying on the one hand, can be some of the most difficult and low months of your life too. Time that was once your own, has suddenly been taken away from you. If you are anything like me, you took for granted the time and space you had to shower, blow dry your hair, choose clothes and accessories for the day ... effortless, peaceful moments in your day. Time you previously had to yourself to recharge, rest, read, workout, catch up with friends, go to the salon or hairdresser, now seldom happens. It can become such a logistical nightmare that you feel it is simply not worth the effort.

However, now that it's not so easy to have "me" time, now is the time you will most need it, and benefit from it. If you don't prioritize this, it will take effect on the inside (felling stressed, irritable, worn-out, etc.) and manifest on the outside too. Most moms automatically put themselves on the bottom of the priority list. Being a mom does require one sacrifice after the next. Well done for all your hard work! The stuff you do all day, every day that can often be left unnoticed ... I know you're doing a super job! But, reality check ... as moms, our labors of love never come to an end, so please don't keep waiting for your needs to get to the top of the list. It is really important that you schedule time to invest in yourself. Looking after yourself *is* loving your child! If you don't, I guess that you will soon suffer from stress; low self esteem, low confidence, and eventually burn out. I want to help you prioritize and organize your life as a young mom so this precious time and role will be something you love and cherish and not a time you simply survive.

Through reading this book I believe you will discover things about yourself that you previously didn't recognize or appreciate. You will realize things about who you are, and how you work best. Your child and partner deserve the best of you, but they too have to help you be your best! It will help to explain to your partner how you love motherhood but how it has dramatically changed the time you have to yourself and how much you feel a little time and space will really help you feel good and maintain a happy positive environment at home for everyone. Let's discover what is most important to you.

Spend some time thinking about what makes you feel:
- Confident
- Happy
- Appreciated
- Attractive
- Alive
- Energetic
- Enthusiastic

Essentially, I want you to invest time and energy in to things that are life giving, and not life sucking! I am going to briefly look at two areas of life that may help shape a positive outlook and help your general well-being.

Get out and be with people!

It can be such an effort to simply leave the house with a young baby you may find yourself opting not to bother. If it seems too difficult and you are hesitant, I want to encourage you to do it! Go for it! The first few times you trip out with your baby without an extra pair of hands to help you can be daunting. Believe me, it does get easier and your confidence will grow. You will learn to not only manage but to thrive on these trips! Meeting with other people, especially other moms who understand what you are going through will encourage and affirm you. The 'people contact' change can be dramatic and have a huge impact on you. Leaving a full time job where you met with people throughout each day, to long days alone with your baby, with limited adult conversation can be both tiresome and confidence wrecking. Make every effort to keep in touch with your long-standing buddies. Go out for coffee during the day or meet for an evening drink. Exercise with friends too as this kills two birds with one stone. Join a club ... do what you can. Sometimes you may have to push yourself to go out when you just don't feel like it. Chances are you won't regret your decision. However, don't neglect rest and good sleep. I remember times when I was literally shaking on an evening because I felt totally exhausted from doing too much! Don't overdo it. Recognize your limits and don't put yourself under too much pressure. Your friends will understand!

Your appearance

How you feel about yourself on the outside greatly affects how you feel on the inside. If you want to feel great on the inside, make an effort to look your best!

Ok, we all have days where we spend less than 60 seconds on our appearance before we walk out the door. In fact I often had a moment of panic that reoccurred on a nearly weekly basis ... I would be on my way somewhere when I suddenly thought I had forgotten to put my jeans on ... the thought of walking down the street in my pants, even for a split moment was horrifying! My heart literally flipped as I looked down to check that I was actually dressed. You know how it is. As moms we have so many things to pack and do before we walk out the door! If you have only a couple of minutes to get yourself ready it helps to only have clothes you love and know you can throw on and feel good in. Get rid of your maternity clothes and the old clothes, and the clothes that don't fit anymore! Otherwise you will waste precious time putting on and taking off, and putting on and taking off clothes!

Wear clothes that fit and look great! Shopping for clothes may now be a different experience to one you were used to. If once you could wear anything and everything and look great, this unfortunately may no longer be the case. Sometimes a woman's body can change shape after pregnancy. I'm thinking hips and breasts!! You now may have to buy clothes that suit your new shape. Discover what looks good now. If you are lucky enough to be without pushchair it will be easier to enjoy shopping and buy the right clothes. Warning: shopping with a baby has its challenges! You have to discover where all the lifts are, where you feel comfortable to breast feed, where you can use bottle warmers/microwaves, where the toilets and changing rooms are in which you can fit in with your pushchair, and find changing facilities for your baby. All this eats away at your shopping time ... be prepared for the shock! Anyhow, despite these challenges it is important you take the time to find clothes you feel comfortable and confident in. Note: finding clothes on trend that you love and can breastfeed in, is time consuming ... good luck to all those who are breastfeeding at a wedding! I'm not trying to be negative here, just realistic.

I believe it is important to treat yourself (see my chapter on motivation) to help you feel good. You deserve it! And as the ad says, "You're Worth It". Do your nails, go have your hair cut, book a shoulder and back massage (if you don't suffer tight shoulders from holding your baby, you must be super woman), go to a spa for a day... ok, so if your reaction is "impossible", new target ... shave your legs! Take pride in your appearance. If you want to look amazing, put the effort in. Do SOMETHING to make yourself feel good about you. Two strategies that will cost you nothing: smile more and stand up straight! Smiling not only makes you look and feel better, it has an impact on others around you. People like to be with those who smile and laugh a lot! They will feel happier when you smile, as happiness is contagious. Actually you will even find that people treat you differently. People who smile more, generally get treated better because others respond positively to the aura this exudes. Try it! Standing up straight is also positive body language. Good posture exudes confidence and is better for you. Poor posture puts pressure on your back and neck and can have knock-on effects of pain and immobility. Who wants to look like a hunch back anyway?

Throughout pregnancy many women are blessed with thick luscious hair and could have modeled for shampoo companies! The bad news ... a few months after giving birth we are often shocked that we begin to lose what seems like a lot of hair! Here's what's going on. Normally, about 85 to 95 per cent of the hair on your head is growing and the other 5 to 15 per cent is in a resting stage. After the resting period, this hair falls out, (often while you're brushing or shampooing) and is replaced by new growth. The average head loses 100 hairs a day, it sounds like a lot but in reality you don't notice it so much. During pregnancy, increased levels of estrogen prolong the growing stage. Therefore, there are fewer hairs in the resting stage and fewer falling out each day, so you have thicker, more luxuriant tresses. After you give birth, your estrogen levels fall and a lot more hair follicles enter the resting stage, causing hair to fall out. The hair that would have normally already have fallen out over the last nine months suddenly falls out, making hair loss pretty noticeable. As a new mom therefore, you now not only have a reduce time for styling, but also don't have natures blessings! However, don't worry! There is light at the end of the plughole! Hair experts say this unusual shedding will taper off and your hair will be back to its pre-pregnancy thickness six to twelve months after you give birth. There are means to help you through this patch.

Top tips for tip top hair

- Keep your hair healthy by eating well and taking a prenatal vitamin supplement (check out chapter 5 on Eating and Drinking).
- Be extra-gentle during your shedding season. Shampoo only when needed, and use a good conditioner and a wide-toothed comb to minimize tangling.
- Use scrunchies instead of rubber bands, and avoid pulling your hair into tight do's.
- Skip blow-drying and straighteners, and put off any chemically based treatments (highlights) until the shedding stops.
- Experiment with different hairstyles or products (such as hair thickeners or

mousse) to give your hair a fuller look during this transition period.

- Avoid stress. Having a new baby to take care of often creates more stress in your life, but endeavor to avoid additional stressful situations as this can affect hair loss and quality.
- Talk to your doctor if your hair loss is excessive and especially if this is coupled with feeling unwell. Hair loss after pregnancy can be a sign of thyroid problems or anemia.

Your skin has undergone significant changes and challenges throughout pregnancy and thus there is a chapter given to detailing this topic. I have included lots of information and advice on how to improve your skin.

Exercise has an unparalleled positive influence on how we look and feel. I am convinced that taking part in exercise will be one of the most beneficial uses of "Me time" for new moms. As 'happy chemicals' are pumped round the body, it will help you simultaneously de-stress and recharge! Furthermore, it will essentially give you back the body you want! Due to the enormity of the effect of exercise there is a whole chapter devoted to this. Dive in!

Chapter 4 - Your Skin

Throughout pregnancy there are so many hormonal changes occurring inside your body it is no surprise that these changes show on the outside, especially in your skin. We all admire perfect complexions. When we see smooth, flawless, dewy skin, we notice! We long for beautiful skin regardless of pregnancy or not. The problem is, attaining complexion perfection after pregnancy can be more difficult than before baby days. Some lucky individuals, the 'glowing' ones, will experience little to no changes in their skin during and after pregnancy, but many will experience several changes. Unfortunately, these are usually changes for the worse, not for the better. The dreaded stretch marks, varicose veins, spider veins, pigmentation, linea nigra, loose skin, chafing, sensitivity, itchiness and dryness ... fear not, most of these skin changes will naturally recover over time. However, there are things you can do to help your skin to be as beautiful as possible once again. If you're reading this during pregnancy, you have an advantage as you can follow my advice and start now in giving your skin its best possible chance! If not, don't worry, start now. If you have bought this book, you care. The chances are you have already been taking care of your skin ... great stuff!

This chapter will cover six of the most common skin problems following pregnancy. I look at what is happening in the body and what we can do to help. There are many websites that list one product or treatment after the next. Most of these are pretty drastic and expensive! There is so much you can do to help improve the condition of your skin, it is not always necessary to undergo such treatment. If you really are concerned about a specific skin condition ensure you do thorough research, see your doctor and seek specialist help before delving in!

Stretch marks! Please ... not me!

Skin specialists suggest that you inherit your mom's skin, and therefore if your mom suffered from stretch marks then you may unfortunately be prone to them too. If not, you are blessed! You may have seen stretch marks appearing as you put on weight during pregnancy. They are slightly discolored purply red streaky lines. They may be hardly noticeable on some, but unfortunately they can be obvious on others. They commonly appear on the middle region, where most of our body shape has changed; your belly, bum, hips and breasts. Pregnancy causes your skin to stretch more and faster than usual. Furthermore, higher levels of hormones also disrupt your skin's protein balance, making it thinner.

Sadly, there's little you can do to prevent stretch marks, but there's plenty you can do to try to minimize them. Be regular and consistent with your regime!

- Avoid putting on too much weight too quickly during pregnancy.
- Massage oil or cream several times a day over the target areas to keep skin supple and elastic and to encourage new tissue growth.
- Eat a healthy diet rich in nutrients. Vitamins E and C, and zinc and silica all help keep your skin healthy.

After pregnancy, the marks should gradually fade and become silvery white in color, and less noticeable. It can take around six months for this to happen.

Dry crocodile skin!

For some women, hormonal changes rob skin of oil and elasticity causing dry, itchy and sometimes flaky skin. Not the best look as well as being rather uncomfortable (I know, I had it).

Because skin is lacking hydration after pregnancy, the sooner you restore moisture levels, the sooner your complexion will return to normal. To help it on its way consider the following:

- Fish oil supplements! Helping from the inside out. Taking these worked wonders for me and within a few weeks my skin felt so, so much better. The itching had disappeared. Happy days!

- A diet including good fats (mono and polyunsaturated), which are found in foods such as olive and canola oils, nuts, and avocados.

- Drink lots of water. Hydration, hydration, hydration!

- Don't wash too much, especially with strong soaps. You could switch to a non soap cleanser to remove make-up before you go to bed, and use only water in the morning.

- Keep showers and baths warm but not steaming hot. Hot water removes natural oil from the skin.

- Slather on moisturizer several times a day, not forgetting your hands too. You could try fragrance-free, additive-free and non-comedogenic for sensitive skin. For especially raw areas, use a hydrating lotion with natural lipids like shea butter or jojoba seed oil.

- Don't be tempted to steam your skin as this can make it increasingly dehydrated.

- Don't rub your skin dry after bathing. Instead lightly pat your skin with a soft towel and apply moisturizer straight away to seal in the water before it has a chance to escape.

Melasma, otherwise known as the "mask of pregnancy"

This is when pigment typically collects around the cheeks, forehead, eyes and sometimes around the mouth. It causes a darkening of skin on lighter-toned faces and lighter patches in the darker skinned. It is caused mainly by UV exposure, however genetics and elevated progesterone levels are also contributing factors. The key to this problem is prevention rather than cure. If you have a history of this condition start to use high protection sunscreen as soon as possible! Is this problem long-term? Specialists suggest that it may clear spontaneously without treatment after pregnancy. Other times, it may clear with sunscreen usage and sun avoidance. For some people, the discoloration may disappear totally, while for others, the discoloration may never completely go away. If you continue to suffer with this after pregnancy you may want to discuss your concerns with your doctor and avoid the use of birth control pills and hormone therapy (HRT) when the time comes!

In order to treat melasma, combination or specially formulated creams with hydroquinone (HQ), a phenolic hypopigmenting agent, azelaic acid, and retinoic acid (tretinoin), nonphenolic bleaching agents, and/or kojic acid may be prescribed. For severe cases of melasma, creams with a higher concentration of HQ or combining HQ with other ingredients such as tretinoin, corticosteroids, or glycolic acid may be effective in lightening the skin. Regular medical follow-up appointments with a doctor are important for people using HQ treatment. Additionally, skin experts say there are many types and strengths of chemical peels available for different skin types. The type of peel should be tailored for each individual and selected by the physician.

Ok, there are a lot of long scientific words here ... but at least you know you can get help! Only pursue this type of treatment, however, if this is really important to you. You may decide not to take this action. If you do decide to go down this path, please make sure you are fully aware of any risks involved and have taken expert advice. If you are still pregnant or breastfeeding you may need to wait to begin this treatment because of possible risks to the developing fetus and newborn. You could consider cosmetic makeup to conceal the skin discoloration!

Loose skin!!

Rapid weight loss following pregnancy can cause skin to sag and appear loose. No more description is needed! You all know what this is. Undeniably, for extreme cases plastic surgery is the most obvious, dramatic and successful way to deal with this problem. However, this is not the best answer for many of us. Your skin may only be slightly loose and not need such drastic measures. You may feel the risks outweigh the benefits, and of course there is the question of financial cost! Fear not! The following fact is not widely advertised: skin is a live organ and can be reshaped and changed, reversing a number of the adjustments it underwent when you were pregnant. There are therefore a number of actions you can take which will contribute to improving the tone of your skin.

8 top ways to tighten your post-pregnancy loose skin!

The best way to maintain elasticity in the skin is to lose your baby weight slowly so that the skin has time to adjust to the reduction in body fat.

Build muscle to fill the skin that has been left behind by body fat loss and birth (see my chapter on exercise).

Keep the skin well moisturized using lotions that contain aloe vera, cocoa butter or soy protein, which will help restore moisture to the skin and encourage collagen and elastin production. Apply moisturizer twice daily and after every shower.

Exfoliate the skin daily in the shower using a scrub or a loofah to remove dead skin cells and increase circulation and cellular growth at the skin surface.

Drink plenty of water to keep the tissues of the body well hydrated. (Dehydration will result in dry skin that appears more wrinkled and saggy).

Nutrition – add raw foods for an antioxidant-rich diet. Simply eat fruit and vegetables raw when you can. In addition to raw foods, eating soy protein will cause your body to produce more collagen, helping skin become taut. See my chapter on nutrition for a more complete explanation and advice on this.

Have a bath! Easy! Taking a bath each week can also help sagging skin. It is said to stimulate circulation, hydrate and detoxify the skin. Add 1/2 pound of sea salt to your bath.

Be patient, time will truly help your skin go back to its normal firmness.

Linea nigra is the Latin for "black line".

Amazingly some women look forward to having this! It is the dark line that appears on the abdomen during many pregnancies, running vertically down the middle of the belly from the belly button (or sometimes higher) to the pubic area. It is caused by an increase in melanocyte, a stimulating hormone made by the placenta. Fair-skinned women show this phenomenon less often than women with darker pigmentation. The line will fade after you give birth. If it still shows slightly, use sun cream protection when your belly is soaking up the rays. Protecting it from UV rays will help it fade over time.

Varicose and spider veins

Many new moms report the appearance of thread veins (often referred to as spider veins). They are most commonly found on the face, chest and legs and are associated with increased levels of estrogen. Varicose and spider veins are hard to prevent but keeping your legs elevated (and not crossed) when you can does help. Wearing compression stockings and exercising regularly can aid too. Specialists advise women to wait at least three to four months following childbirth before embarking on major treatment as they often go away without intervention. However, if they don't, they can be treated in various medical ways, the best course of action dependent on their severity and location.

Having looked at the most common effects pregnancy has on skin I want to remind you that beauty is not just skin deep. Don't be too harsh and critical of yourself when you look at your skin. Your body has paid a price for having a baby ... but it was worth it! You have made a baby ... a friend for life! Keep motivated, do your best, follow my guidelines, work hard but be patient.

Just a note...

If you smoked before and stopped for pregnancy, well done! Now stay off the cigarettes! Do not rebuild the habit. Find other means of stress relief or escapism that does not wreck your skin's ability to recover and rejuvenate. Smoking is damaging to your hair and teeth too, both of which have an obvious impact on the way you look. Your beauty will glow brighter without the cigarettes!

Chapter 5 - Food and Drink

Food is more than simply fuel for our bodies and fuel to supply our baby with milk. Food is a part of community, building relationships, sharing, nurturing, celebrating and having fun together. It is something that is a huge part of life. Without it, we would miss out on so much. I really am so grateful for food. I love it. Sometimes the taste is exquisite and luxurious, other times simply warm, friendly, filling and satisfying. I have known food to even bring adventure, giving rise to anticipation and excitement. I love food not only for what it is, but for the moments in life it brings friends and families together and for the memories it creates. Food is not just good, it's great!

Throughout life there are times and seasons where people naturally either lose weight and decrease body fat, or put on weight and increase body fat. For example, during the summer season we naturally eat more salads and lighter foods, and exercise more whist enjoying the outdoors. This leads to weight loss. In contrast the winter season is notorious for indulging in party food both at work and at home. Friends and family gather for numerous celebrations at Christmas and New Year. We comfort eat while we stay, sitting, indoors during the long dark cold evenings.

Moving house can be a period in life that leads to weight loss due to high stress levels, busyness in packing, unpacking and tackling DIY projects. Life events, such as family weddings (your own or someone else's) may be a motivation to eat well in order to feel good and fit into the dress we desire on that special day. In contrast, pregnancy is a time in life where women (and often even their partners) put on weight. This weight gain and even the increased body fat is normal, natural and healthy for pregnant women. But sadly, many women struggle to ever lose this weight gain and often, with each child a few pounds (or more) is added.

This weight gain is understandable. We live in a society where there is
ever available food around us. Unfortunately after having a baby we live with added opportunities and temptations and reasons why we may overeat or simply consistently consume the wrong types of food.

Prior to having your baby you were generally more active in the evenings. You spent many evenings out of the house, be it going for evening strolls, or to the gym or to exercise classes, social gatherings, pursuing hobbies, or even shopping. Having had a baby and wanting to be there for him, we now stay in the house most evenings, most likely sitting watching the TV or reading, or surfing the internet. There is nothing wrong with this. In many ways you do need to simply rest. However it does mean you are less active and have time to pass...and so we reach for the snacks. Simply a way to pass time. A little like when you are on a long journey, there is nothing else to do, so you eat. This can be especially so when we are home alone with no other adult company and even more so if we feel lonely and isolated.

You may feel that you deserve to overindulge in food...you have just made a baby, endured delivery and worked hard all day looking after the new arrival. You **do** deserve a reward, I'm just not sure this is the best type of reward!

The first few weeks after delivery are often busy with close friends and family visiting and if they don't bring biscuits, cake and chocolate with them, you are more than likely to feel you should provide this for them to celebrate the new baby together. I'm guessing a lot expectant parents fill their cupboards with delicious sweet treats to bring out for celebrating with friends and family visitors. Aware of the challenge ahead and lack of time to bake any homemade treats, you prepare the cupboards. Mmmmm, there is always going to be biscuits left on the plate when everyone has gone. ...

When the initial celebratory weeks have passed, you begin to join in community activities that bring young moms and their babies and toddlers together. Believe me, there are always biscuits involved. Opportunities galore!

It is not uncommon for new moms to have low self-esteem. The extra weight gained, the skin damage, the tired eyes, the old misshaped and unflattering clothes ... it is easy to understand why a combination of theses factors can easily have a negative impact on self esteem. Alas, low self-esteem can often lead to taking less care of yourself and comfort eating.

Simply believing you now have to eat for two can encourage over consumption of calories. You feel hungry due to breastfeeding, or feel tired and lacking in energy so you continuously snack to top yourself up. You simply feel you need the energy boost to get the jobs done you need to.

As a busy mom you will probably find you have less time to cook homemade food from scratch. Not only is the cooking too demanding time wise, but the physical act of going to the supermarket with your baby is daunting, never mind finding the time and inspiration you need to plan the shopping list. Due to such challenges you may get takeaway or ready-meals more than you have ever done before.

I do understand all these reasons (and there are plenty more) for eating, but I do want to encourage you to take a few moments whilst reading this chapter to try and challenge yourself and think about the food choices you are making. What is the impact these choices are having on your health and well-being, and what impact this will have on your new family. I want the best for you and your growing family and I know you do too.

Nutrition is a massive subject in itself, and would require book after book to cover all the ins and outs of the best types of diet and still then it is hard to find a diet that actually works well and consistently with life. In this one chapter I want to highlight key principles, and look at some of the fundamentals of understanding food and healthy eating, especially relating this to new moms. I will cover important topics such as consuming alcohol and caffeine, supplementation, hydration, meals to aid healing and recovery after delivery, nutrition for breastfeeding, healthy snacking, calorie consumption and losing weight.

There are so many conflicting messages, and philosophies on diets that it can be a point of tension, but I want to present my underlining belief that food is to be enjoyed. In the developed world we're privileged to access unlimited amounts of food and an unbelievably wide variety of choice! Lets enjoy this, without taking it for granted and without becoming over indulgent. After all, a treat is not a treat when it becomes the norm!

I'm presenting the beliefs and principles that I currently hold. This however does not mean that they won't change and evolve over time. As scientific literature develops and expands I will continue to learn more and I expect my understanding and life application will develop. I will provide you information that will help you make informed choices. I will not bog you down with complicated scientific mechanisms, but simply present information and offer guidelines and practical help. All of which is underpinned by years of reading, extensive research and information, discussing with experts, personal experience and also the valuable experiences of many friends who have been through pregnancy and entered the world of babies and toddlers!

Drinks

We are 70% water. We need to constantly replenish this vital nutrient, unadulterated and clean. Its functions are varied—filtering, cleansing, moistening, lubricating, supporting and transporting. A majority of what you drink should be water. However, I know this is more of a challenge for some than others. Depending on where you live, the taste of tap water varies greatly. For those people who live in areas where the water tastes good it is easier to drink. For those who live in an area where the taste of water is not so nice have probably got used to drinking very little water. You have probably got used to buying squash's or fruit juices to dilute with water in order to mask its unpleasant taste. This habit comes with warning. Doing this adds many useless calories. It would be worth considering simply buying bottled spring water, which would be of similar financial cost but without the extra calories. Forming a new habit of drinking water will act as a great example to your baby, to be toddler, when they begin drinking from a cup or beaker. If toddlers constantly sip on juice throughout the day it will prove extremely damaging for their teeth as well as causing frequent sugar spikes in their body. It is always the best example to a child when you practice what you speak.

Drinking plenty is of the upmost importance when you are breastfeeding. Amazingly, the body is good at telling you what it needs. Many moms, whilst breastfeeding actually feel thirsty during a feed. Most moms set themselves up with a huge pint glass or sports bottle next to them during a feed. You really do need it!

If drinking water does seem completely unappealing try to be creative with your drinks. Rather than having coffee after coffee or fruit juice followed by fruit juice, explore the huge variety of herbal teas. Some herbal teas can even help with problems you maybe facing. For example, some aid digestion, others promote calm before sleep. Popular teas include mint tea, licorice tea and Rooibos. One of the drinks I most enjoyed having while breastfeeding was my pint sized mid morning protein shake. I also loved a milk shake or two. Be adventurous and try new drinks.

Fruit juice
(Bought fruit juice and juicing fruit at home)

Drinking fruit juices can benefit health as you absorb vitamins and minerals from the fruit, however a downside of juicing is that you often lose out on the goodness found in the skin and pith. Secondly, because there is a lot of fruit in just one glass there is also a lot of sugar (even if it is natural sugar), and therefore calories too. This becomes a definite problem when someone is trying to loose weight.

If you need to drink fruit juices to consume liquid, it would be better to dilute it with water. The high sugar content in straight fruit juice spikes your insulin levels, which soon drop, making you feel hungry and wanting to eat again. Diluting the juice would also help avoid the effect straight fruit juice has on increasing your blood cholesterol.

If however you are drinking fruit juice as an energy drink during a work out, this will work well, providing a high-energy boost.

Alcohol

I'm sorry to say it is best to keep alcohol down to a minimum if you are breastfeeding. After nine months of pretty much abstinence during my pregnancies (I literally had a sip here and there that tasted divine!) I really wanted to enjoy treating myself to a glass of wine at the weekends. Many sources suggest that you should not drink alcohol at all during the months of breastfeeding. However, if you decide to drink some alcohol while feeding, experts suggest drinking after a feed and not just before. Looking on the bright side, abstinence will help your calorie intake to remain lower if you are trying to loose the extra weight you may have gained during pregnancy (an average glass of wine is 250 calories).

Caffeine

Many popular drinks such as filter coffee, cappuccinos, lattes and tea contain caffeine. These drinks like food, I believe are here to be enjoyed! Young parents often reach out for such drinks at a time in life when they are in need of a quick pick-me-up both mentally and physically. Caffeine improves cognitive performance; reaction time and short term recall ... all areas where new parents appreciate an occasional boost! The night before an important day at work may have been tough, leaving you feeling rather frazzled, blurry and slow. We all know a strong coffee can help.

There are further benefits to coffee too. It contains beneficial antioxidants, methylpyridinium being the most well known one. According to the latest studies on the subject, moderate coffee consumption seems to be protective against cardiovascular disease. It also seems to offer protection to the liver and has been found to reduce the incidence of liver cancer.

To many people, coffee is not only absolutely delicious but also proves a great way to stay on track with a diet helping individuals from indulging in other unhealthy choices. Coffee stimulates peristalsis and can help those who suffer from constipation. This could be useful information for those who may struggle going to the toilet soon after giving birth.

Unfortunately caffeine does have its down sides too. However, these down sides mainly occur with over consumption and dependency on caffeine, rather than within moderate consumption. These are just a few factors to be aware of:

- New parents have already had their **sleep** patterns drastically altered with the new little arrival, and caffeine may lead to further sleep disturbances.

- Coffee **hinders iron absorption** due to its tannin content. It can therefore further exacerbate iron deficiency. Following pregnancy some women need to be aware of this and alter caffeine consumption.

- We do know that some of the caffeine (around 1%) that a breastfeeding mom consumes can get through into **breast milk**. However, we do not know the exact effect this caffeine has on the baby. Some experts suggest this will have very little effect. Others argue that due to the fact that a baby can struggle to get rid of caffeine in their blood stream, a build up may occur. This can lead to a baby being wakeful, restless or irritable. Therefore, if your baby struggles to settle to sleep or wakes up often, or generally seems unsettled or restless, you could try cutting down on your caffeine consumption or even cutting it out completely. A good friend of mine was struggling with her 6 month old baby waking several times a night despite the fact that the baby was not hungry. My friend then decided to cut out caffeine to see if this had an effect. From the second night onwards her baby slept through! I figure it is worth a try. A simple solution to a difficult situation.

Caffeine occurs naturally in coffee, tea and cocoa, used in chocolate, but be aware that caffeine is also added to soft drinks, energy drinks and is even in cold and flu remedies.

As mentioned earlier, it is important to drink plenty but try a variety of drinks to avoid consuming lots of caffeine. Try de-caffeinated tea and coffee, herbal teas, heavily diluted fruit juice (10:1 i.e. 10 parts of water to 1 part of juice), milk shakes and protein shakes (check these as some types contain caffeine).

As a general guideline, if you are going to drink caffeinated drinks in moderation, limit filter coffee consumption to two cups a day and tea to four cups per day.

Food and meals that will help with healing

Preparation for recovery begins right back before pregnancy begins. Eating a healthy diet before conception builds up nutrient reserves for you and your growing baby. Continuing to eat healthily during pregnancy is essential for your postnatal recovery and breastfeeding as well as for your baby's growth and development. Your baby receives its nutrition not only from what you eat but also from your body's reserves. Therefore, if you are not eating well before and during pregnancy, your body may suffer. The good news is that you can prepare your body for a speedy recovery well in advance of the baby arriving and before life gets a whole lot busier. If you are reading this after giving birth, don't worry, there is still plenty you can do to help your body recover well. Here are a few top tips:

- The key is to 'keep it simple and avoid processed junk'! Food should be fresh, seasonal and organic if possible. Eat a wide range of foods to get a wide range of nutrients.

- Stock up the freezer before labor with nutritious, home-cooked meals.

- Have a collection of quick, healthy recipes to hand for you or someone offering to cook for you. If you have an extended hospital stay, why not ask friends to bring in salads and fruit.

Have a stock of healthy snacks available to eat at home, and to take with you when you leave the house (see below for ideas)

Here are a few simple meals:

These foods and meals will help with healing and recovery soon after delivery.

Salmon, new potatoes, organic crème fraîche with fresh watercress

Wholegrain pasta, pesto, organic chicken and broccoli

Wholegrain rice, omelet and vegetables lightly stir-fried in coconut oil

Baked sweet potatoes, hummus and salad

It is a great idea to have plenty of healthy **snacks** on hand too.

Snacks

Sourdough rye bread with nut butter and banana

Fruit and organic cheese e.g. cheddar and grapes, cream cheese and apple slices

Whole meal pitta and hummus

Veggies such as carrots, peppers, cucumber (cutting them into handy sticks works well), cherry tomatoes and sugar snaps.

Dried fruit, nuts and seeds (apricots are high in iron, figs high in digestive enzymes, and prunes are great for reducing constipation)

Oatcakes (these come in all different flavors) and cheese

Boiled eggs (full of nutrients for healing and recovery, brain function and energy)

Olives

Red bell pepper dipped in guacamole

Handful of strawberries with 2 squares of dark chocolate

Sliced tomato sprinkled with herbs and feta or chunks of mozzarella

Flaked coconut and dates

Natural Greek yoghurt with raspberries or honey

Eating healthy food is the best way to get all the nutrients your body needs. However, before, during and after pregnancy, your body needs extra help. If you have a continued diet of hospital food or are exhausted and barely have energy to eat, let alone prepare a healthy meal, your body needs good quality supplements to help boost recovery. It would be useful to buy a couple of pill organizers for your hospital bag and to keep at home afterwards. This helps you remember which supplements you have taken when all your days and nights tend to blur into one!

Supplements

- A good quality **multivitamin** and mineral supplement (if you are breastfeeding make sure it is recommended for this). You can keep taking your prenatal vitamins but make sure they include **iron** to build up reserves following any blood loss. Iron also aids in wound healing and helps protect against infection. Ensure **calcium** is present too, for bone strength, and **zinc** for wound healing and which also can help lower the effects of postnatal depression and promote healthy hormones.

- **1000mg Vitamin C** with bioflavonoids – this is great for wound healing, iron absorption, skin repair and helping prevent postnatal depression and infection.

- **Fish oils** – may help healing and skin repair, lower inflammation, improve sleep, boost energy, reduce afterbirth pains, nourish your brain (most moms suffer from 'mommy brain' at some point!) and lower the chances of postnatal depression.

- **Vitamin D3** – may decrease the risk of pre-eclampsia, gestational diabetes, pre-term delivery and high blood pressure for the mother and may decrease the risk of asthma, low birth weight and heart disease for the baby. It is recommended that you take a minimum of 400iu, but many experts recommend up to 4000iu both during and after pregnancy.

- **Glutamine** – may help with the healing of soft tissue, especially following a caesarean (as long as you have no liver problems). Take this as a supplement for the first 2 weeks and then just eat glutamine rich foods such as eggs, beef, chicken, yoghurt, milk, cottage cheese, ricotta cheese, spinach and cabbage.

- **Vitamin E oil** – may help reduce the appearance of stretch marks and scars (once the wound has healed) and improve skin condition. Try piercing a vitamin E capsule with a pin and rubbing the oil directly onto the skin.

- **Coconut oil** – may help to improve your skin after birth. Apply directly to the skin.

Nutrition and breastfeeding

Is there anything I can do nutritionally to improve my breast milk? Many moms ask this question, sometimes in desperation! At times we feel we are not producing enough milk for our baby and are keen to boost our supply to keep baby satisfied. Others, simply want to ensure they are doing all they can to give their baby the best start in life possible.

This is a huge topic and there have been some excellent books written about this subject. The simple answer is yes. There are certain foods that can help boost the quality and quantity of your milk!

Adapting your diet to improve your milk supply

- **Phytoestrogens** – these are thought to boost lactation by stimulating the growth of milk-glands in the breast. Oats, millet, barley, rice, chickpeas, peas, lentils, green beans and quinoa are all rich in phytoestrogens. Soaking or sprouting the grains makes them more digestible. You can soak muesli or oats overnight before having them for breakfast.

- **Saponins** – these can influence the body's ability to make lactation hormones. Foods rich in saponins include oats, asparagus, chickpeas and potatoes with their skins on.

- **Serotonin** – this helps your body to relax and feel good which is essential for lactation. Your body makes serotonin from tryptophan. Great sources of tryptophan are almonds, cashews, pecans, sesame and flax seeds.

- **Natural sedatives** – certain foods have a sedating effect which increases prolactin in your body, increasing the production of breast milk. Good foods to eat are lettuce, onion, fennel and potato.

- **Oils and fats** – these are essential for quality and quantity of breast milk. Good oils are cold-pressed nut and seed oils (keep them in the fridge), butter, coconut oil and olive oil. Some people recommend taking 3-4tbsp of coconut oil per day, and that supplementing vitamin D boosts milk supply too. Worth a try!

Things which can reduce milk production:

There are a few things to be aware of which can reduce milk production:

- **Dieting and calorie restriction** – can reduce the quantity and nutritional content of a mother's milk. Sudden weight loss may also cause toxins to be released into the breast milk. Breastfeeding, on the other hand can help to get rid of fat deposits in your body.
- **Caffeine** – foods such as chocolate, tea and coffee may reduce milk supply by inhibiting the let-down reflex and causing the constriction of capillaries in the breast.
- **Herbs** – parsley, rosemary, peppermint, thyme, spearmint and lemon balm may reduce the supply of breast milk.
- **Vitamin C** – excessive amounts of vitamin C either as supplements or eating lots of citrus fruits may reduce milk supply
- **Vitamin B6** (pyridoxine) – over 200mg a day may reduce milk supply.
- **Bananas, apples and avocados** – while they are great foods to eat in moderation, if eaten in excess they may inhibit milk production in some women.
- **Aspartame** – this is a common sweetener often found in soft drinks, chewing gum,

and 'low sugar' foods. It may reduce milk supply.
- **Over-hydration** – while mothers are encouraged to drink plenty while breastfeeding since you do need slightly more hydration, drinking too much may actually reduce your milk supply. The key is to drink when you are thirsty and stop when your thirst is quenched. For the same reasons, mothers who have an IV drip during labor can have initial challenges with breastfeeding. If this is the case, you should see a breastfeeding counselor for help.

Fat loss

Diet plays a key role in your body composition. In some ways your diet affects the way your body looks more than the exercise you undertake.   I've met significantly overweight people who exercise, but I've never met someone who watches their diet and eats cleanly who is significantly overweight. However, do not lapse in to a false sense of security thinking you do not need to exercise! I said nutrition is a bigger factor than exercise, not that exercise has little effect. It is essential that you give your time and energy to both. I do not promote a good diet and exercise simply to help people look good. It's about feeling good and being healthy too. For example, you can get a slim girl who looks good in skinny jeans yet can be greatly lacking in energy, has bad skin, has no muscle tone, has too much fat deposited around her arteries, is prone is osteoporosis, has a weak heart (remember this is a muscle so you need to work it hard for it to become stronger) and is basically unhealthy. Without exercise supporting a balanced nutritious diet you will not look or feel great.

Unfortunately, statistics show that a majority of women weigh heavier and have an increased body fat in the following months and even years after pregnancy. I believe women would not only look better but would also be healthier, happier and more energetic, leading to a positive impact on their family life too if they managed to regain their previous size and weight. The task of loosing this baby weight is possible!

Firstly, we must recognize that you should not do this too quickly. Extreme dieting and rapid weight loss can be hazardous to your health. A new mom should initially focus on recovery and health rather than weight loss. It takes 9 months to grow a baby and can take 9 months to a year to recover and build up your nutritional reserves again. Rapid weight loss can even affect your metabolism leading to long term weight gain. Focusing on regaining your health and eating well helps you to get back to a healthy weight in a sensible way. It would also help set a good example for your baby as they wean and begin to eat meals. Secondly, significant calorie restriction should only be done after finishing breastfeeding and not before. Breast feeders ... do not despair, there is hope. Fat loss will occur if you follow a healthy eating program. When I say breastfeeding moms should not be on a calorie restricted diet, this is not a license to overeat or choose foods that will put on weight or which are 'empty calories'. This is a time in life when you should put extra time and thought in to your nutritional input as you do have reserves to replenish and a baby to nourish. This will not be accomplished on a diet of sweets, cola, cakes and biscuits! Following a healthy eating program will help to decrease your body fat, despite not being on a calorie restricted diet. In fact gradual weight loss over several months is the safest and most effective way to lose body fat. Breastfeeding moms actually have an advantage in the fact they are burning 200-500 extra calories a day! Furthermore, research reveals that breastfeeding actually helps burn fat! All moms, following birth will immediately lose about 10lbs or more of weight, plus a little more as fluid decreases over the first few days. Everyone has this initial weight loss! Following the birth of my third son I remember feeling like the slimmest, lightest woman in the world ... quite untrue having gained four stone (over 25Kgs!) throughout pregnancy, but it was a good start!

Healthy Eating Principles
(This is not wishy washy...it changes lives)

Eat **REAL food** not FAKE food – don't go on any crazy diets – low fat, low carb, low calorie etc.

Your postnatal body needs real food. By this I mean no processed food, ready meals, instant meals or jars with a huge list of ingredients on them. Eating real food doesn't need to be time consuming. Many new moms I know use a slow cooker, packing loads of vegetables in there. This cuts down shopping time and cooking time and allows you to return home after a day filled with toddler groups, trips to the park and school runs, and sit straight down to a delicious home cooked meal. The more simple and 'real' your food is, the easier it is for your baby to eventually move on to the food you eat which then cuts down the separate meals you have to cook for them.

I'm not keen on cutting out big groups of food unless you are being treated for a specific allergy, condition, or sickness that you're trying to overcome. Cutting out a whole food type, for example potatoes, or carbs, or meat can create problems. Apart from the fact it can be difficult socially, meals are likely to become both bland and lacking in variety and therefore lacking in essential ingredients. Instead of cutting out a major food type or ingredient, try keeping the meal exactly the same but cutting down the **portion size**. That way you eat a gourmet meal without overeating. For some reason, people think that "cooking a lovely meal" is a license to overeat. Why not enjoy the "lovely meal" and leave feeling satisfied but not stuffed!

Eat Full Fat

Yes, this is not a typing error, I said eat full fat. Fat free or low fat normally means high sugar, or added sweeteners and added chemicals to try to make them taste good (not that successfully). These additives are not great for you. Remember, fat in foods such as yogurt, cheese, butter, milk, cream, nuts and olive oil is good fat and is not to be avoided. Eating fat is not bad for you; wearing fat is what is bad for you. In many cases it is the high sugar content in people's diets that cause fat gain and which cause high cholesterol. Interestingly, abdominal fat is linked almost exclusively to refined sugar consumption, the biggest culprits being modified fructose (found in low fat yoghurts and other low fat foods). Studies have revealed that eating fat can actually lower cholesterol! Furthermore, countless examples exist of individuals who move from a low fat diet to a higher fat, lower starch and sugar diet and achieve a much lower body fat AND are able to maintain it. Full fat dairy products are so tasty and so filling. Give it go! When I began changing from low fat to full fat I know I became leaner.

The fat you do need to avoid is trans fat which is found in foods such as pastries, crisps, doughnuts, bought cookies, margarine and ready made meals. These are manmade fats from vegetables oils that have been partially hydrogenated. Trans fat has been shown to increase blood levels of low density lipoprotein (LDL), known as "bad" cholesterol, and lower levels of high density lipoprotein (HDL), or "good" cholesterol. It has numerous effects on our health, which include the major clogging of arteries, type 2 diabetes, increase in the risk of heart disease, and other serious health problems.

Of all the foods available, **protein** has the greatest effect on your metabolism ... it speeds it up! I believe you should eat protein at every meal. Eating foods high in protein, (such as eggs, dairy products, chicken, lentils, nuts) helps you feel fuller for much longer, controlling those hunger pangs. And if you do feel hungry between meals, eating snacks which are high in protein work wonders. While I was breastfeeding I drank a delicious protein shake each day which provided the protein without many calories. Having these shakes stopped me from reaching for other snacks, often which were high in sugar. I felt really satisfied. Many people are aware that protein is needed for growth and repair but do not realize how this is important. Apart from continuous growth and repair functions going on in the body at a cellular level, moms need protein for:

Repair – you have either been through a natural delivery or have had a caesarean, both of which have caused pretty extensive damage to the body and therefore much healing needs to take place.

Growth – protein is actually vital to weight loss as it helps to build and shape those fat burning muscles that burn calories even when you're watching TV. Without sufficient protein these muscles will not grow and develop.

I am not advocating a super high protein diet, but I would say somewhere from 1.7-2.0grams per kilogram bodyweight per day.

Eat Vegetables!

Without a doubt one of the most useful but underrated, underused nutritional strategies is consuming lots of vegetables. Eat as many vegetables as you want. They will fill you up, they will provide the nutrients and vitamins you need for a balanced, healthy diet, and they will not increase your body fat. Broccoli, spinach, lettuce, peppers, cabbage, kale, carrots, leeks, beetroot, bok choy, peas, sweat potato, watercress, asparagus ... keep it varied and colorful. Different colors represent different nutrients!

Plan your meals and plan your food shopping.

If you find it difficult to plan meals, buy some recipe books for inspiration and guidance. Enjoy shopping and be creative. Try foods you have never eaten before! However, don't feel bad if you repeat meals from week to week. Children often find meals they really enjoy and they do not get bored of them. Find what meals work for you and your family and rest in the knowledge you are providing good nutritious food. If you live in an area covered by a supermarket delivery service, why not try this out. It can be a lifesaver in the first few months of having a baby especially if you have a toddler and the new baby to manage whilst shopping. The first few on line shops can take a while, but it gets a lot quicker as you continue to return to the site. Such websites are often simple and easy to understand and follow. The sites have ways of remembering your previous orders, and even show the same offers on products that you would find in the stores!

Freeze meals

Freeze meals for busy times so you can eat good food when you haven't had time to give food a thought. This becomes less important as your child gets older. Although, when you have a number of children, you may find that you continue doing this from time to time. When I have time on my hands I often apply this method and cook a large batch of something to freeze in several portions (for example Bolognese). During busy days when my 3 hungry boys can't wait 45 minutes for the meal to be prepared, or when I am too tired to cook dinner, I can defrost something and still know that I'm giving them something nutritious and tasty. If I know that there is a particularly busy time coming up, I will prepare a few meals in advance. Most often I simply prepare a double quantity of that day's meal. We eat one, and freeze one. I would do this a few times to build up a store. I really appreciate these meals when they appear on the table! They somehow taste better too as I haven't given my time and energy cooking, smelling and tasting throughout the process! It's the next best thing to being cooked for.

Spice your food well

Spices and herbs carry very few calories. Making your food taste good will help you enjoy eating. It's a ludicrous misconception that healthy food tastes bad. Try avoiding bought dressings as they contain sugars and trans fat that promote fat storage. Rather, make your own tasty dressings and marinades with vinegar, olive oil, salt, pepper and other herbs and spices.

Sit down at a table to eat

Doing this prevents mindless snacking on something you can grab instantly which is most likely unhealthy and you won't remember eating or tasting a minute after you have eaten it! It also helps your digestion to be more efficient and get the best out of your food. It sets a good example to your child about mealtimes being relaxed, social and purposeful times to enjoy good food. Generally by always sitting down to eat you end up eating less but enjoying food more.

Have a "cheat day"!

Being relaxed everyday and going with the flow doesn't work. Listening to your body doesn't work. Long term, extreme diets don't work. Having a cheat day does. It is simple, but effective. Traditionally the concept comes from bodybuilders who take cheat days where they can eat anything they want. Any food and any quantity! I like this concept and have used it effectively at different times (actually most of the time). In essence, a cheat day is when you follow an eating plan all week (for me this is simply eating fresh food, whilst avoiding all sugary desserts, soft drinks and crisps) and then eat what you want one day a week. You may want to have a cheat day less frequently. However, it's a great way of being able to reward yourself to treats you might like, enjoy a meal out, and simply relax and go with the flow. Adopting this 'rule' really helps you keep on your eating plan in two main ways:

Firstly it helps to make you feel that you are not depriving yourself...you can have that cake...just not today. When you feel you constantly deprive yourself of treats and you see no end in sight to this, it is easy to give up and give in to your momentary desires. This only leads on to a downward spiral. When you can tell yourself "I can have that in 'x' days time", saying no becomes so much easier. And when your cheat day arrives ... if you still fancy that pudding or cake you wanted earlier in the week, you can have it!

Secondly, it eventually builds a new habit of healthy eating. You will actually enjoy the treat you choose and savor it, after all you have waited for it! Having a cheat becomes actually that. When the norm is to have a sweet treat everyday, it is not actually something special. It has become the norm and what your body expects.

The rationale behind a cheat day is that you cannot consume enough 'bad stuff' in one day to be detrimental to your goal. This is much better than being fairly good all the time, but allowing yourself one treat per day, for example. By doing this, your body never stabilizes its insulin, and the entire knock on processes of eating the right stuff to boost your metabolism does not happen. It takes a certain diet, a certain way of eating, to achieve the metabolic changes, and stabilization that is required for maintaining a good body composition. By being strict with your diet 6 days and week and relaxing for 1 day, you cannot do too much damage and undo the balance that you've achieved, as long as on the eight day you return to your structured, healthy eating.

The cheat day method is also good for those who have a tendency to become legalistic or extremist. Sometimes constant discipline can get out of control and become obsessive and lead to disordered eating.

For those on a controlled diet for a certain

medical condition, for example, due to food intolerance or allergy, cheat days do not work. These special diets require total avoidance of certain ingredients for a certain length of time. These kinds of diets work by starving your body of certain foods that are not good for it, or which it cannot cope with. Therefore, complete abstinence is needed in order to allow the body to heal. In such cases, cheat days break down the whole process of healing and equilibrium and are counterproductive.

Cut down on the white stuff

A diet high in sugar leads to weight gain, heart disease and type 2 diabetes. If that is not hard hitting enough, it also causes premature ageing, tooth decay, mood swings, energy lows and obesity. Recent scientific research even claims it is responsible for Alzheimer's disease and cataracts. Serious stuff. So why don't people suffering with such conditions simply cut right back on sugar consumption? The answer is addiction. Sugar is addictive and the body reacts to it like a drug, craving it constantly. The average Briton consumes 238 teaspoons of sugar a week. Scary! I believe much of this sugar is not knowingly consumed as it is often hidden in foods, drinks and sauces. To give you an idea; a typical bottle of cola or similar soft drink contains 17 cubes of sugar, 1 medium glass of cranberry juice contains 7 cubes, and 150g pot of low fat fruit yogurt 5 cubes. Often it is difficult to understand the information on labels. For example, contents are given in grams of carbohydrate and it is difficult to know what that means in reality. To give you some help 39g in a can of cola is equivalent to 10 cubes of sugar, 65g in a 590 ml bottle of cola is equivalent to 17 cubes, and 108g in a 1 liter sized bottle, 27 cubes.

Food labels actually contain two pieces of information which you need to be able to understand and interpret. There is a table that shows the number of grams of proteins, carbohydrates and fats (macronutrients) in the food. The label shows the number of grams of these macronutrients per 100g of content. This alone, however, is not enough to understand the nutritional composition of the food. For example, a label may indicate 40g of carbohydrate per 100g. If this 40g comes from rice or potato or any other land grown crop, then generally it is okay. If this 40g comes from refined sugar or fructose syrup, for example, then it is extremely high in sugar and should be avoided! Learning to read the **lists of ingredients** on packaged food helps understand where the grams of proteins, carbohydrates and fats really come from. Ingredients are key.

One of the biggest problems with consuming lots of sugar is that **the body easily converts excess sugar into fat**. Any time we have extra sugar in the body, the body absorbs it into the cells or the liver, where it gets converted into fat. In other forms of carbohydrates (such as vegetables and other natural forms), sugar (energy) is released slowly in to the blood stream and is taken and used as the body needs. When refined sugars are consumed, blood sugar levels are quickly raised. The levels spike so high that the body does not need the energy, thus it is turned in to fat. The secondary effect of this sugar spike is that your body is confused in to thinking that it needs these excessive levels of sugar and therefore develops a craving. The only way to satisfy this craving is by consuming more sugar. As a result the body quickly develops a sugar addiction. This is an on going cycle of overconsumption that leads to fat storage. Consuming slow release carbohydrates (low GI foods) avoids such blood sugar spikes and therefore is extremely beneficial to those who want to avoid increases in body fat.

Chapter 6 - Exercise and Activity

Do NOT skip over this chapter! Don't even think about it. Don't be scared. This is a key chapter to engage with if you want that amazing body! It is not written for the already super fit athletes. It is written for you! You can begin to exercise! You can become fit! You can even be super fit! You can change your body! Everyone has to start somewhere, and here is that place. ...

I'm going to look at the benefits of exercise and explain the different types of exercise and what they do for the body. I am also going to highlight key principles to be aware of following pregnancy. Most importantly I'm going to explain exactly what exercises you can do from the very first few days as a new mom through the following weeks and months and beyond. Also included are specific guidelines for those who have had a caesarean section. This chapter is going to motivate you and give you clear, realistic and achievable means to gain that super body you want. I'm even going to give you specific exercises that will completely change the way your body looks. It is simple and it works! Fortunately, alongside my own knowledge, I am able to draw on my husband's 12 years experience working with professional athletes, making sure their bodies are healthy, strong, fast and toned. As a Strength and

Conditioning expert, he is someone who knows about exercise and the human body. I am 100% confident you are going to get the best advice you can possibly get.

Let's consider the benefits of exercise

There are many well-documented benefits of exercise. These are worth reviewing in order to remind us that these advantages are broader than simply looking good! Overviewing the benefits of exercise will definitely fuel our level of motivation.

Here are some of the benefits:

- Promotes weight loss
- Improves your cardiovascular fitness
- Improves muscle strength
- Reduces risk of heart disease
- Reduces risk of diabetes
- Increases bone mineral density i.e. stronger bones, and therefore reduces risk of post menopausal osteoporosis
- Increases capacity for daily tasks i.e. increased stamina
- Improves body function i.e. coordination and strength, which improve the ability to perform physical tasks (note that the capacity for daily tasks and ability to perform daily tasks are not the same thing).
- Lowers health bills

- Strengthens immunity (immediately post exercise, your immune system is suppressed, however, in the long term, you will have a much stronger resistance to sickness and diseases).
- De-stressing effect
- Improves your mood
- Helps prevent and promote recovery from postpartum depression

Types of exercise

There are lots of ways to exercise. Most of which are not particularly right or wrong, but some methods are more *effective* than others. Some people have different preferences too. My general philosophy is to exercise for physical and mental health and longevity, and therefore I chose to do a wide variety of fun activities, alongside a few fundamental aspects that I regard as essential (these can be fun too). It is true that if you are training to run a marathon, you need to run lots. If you are training for a triathlon, you need to include lots of swimming, cycling and running. However, if your focus is to recover from pregnancy and for general fitness, health and happiness, then this chapter is perfect, revealing how best to accomplish this. It will also shortcut your way to having that amazing body you want!

#1 – Include weight training in your program

Incorporating some form of weight training is one of the keys to great health *and* looking good. An increase in muscle mass will increase your metabolism and thus increase the body's fat burning capabilities. Note that 1lb of muscle in your body burns around 50 calories per day (doing nothing, just living!) In comparison, 1lb of fat burns only about 4 calories per day. Therefore if you have more muscle you will be burning off significantly more calories throughout each and every day. Eventually this calorie burning process burns off excess fat. Weight training will also give you a better body shape. Contrary to what many believe, you will not look larger or "chunky" by increasing muscle mass. In fact you will look leaner as your body proportions will be more balanced.

There are many benefits of weight training, some of which are listed above in the benefits of general exercise. I would also like to highlight some specific benefits of weight training which impact how you look and feel:

- Stronger body
- Increased metabolism (increased fat burning capabilities)
- Reduced risk of injury (stronger muscles and joints)
- Reduced risk of heart disease and diabetes
- Better balance and coordination

@ Better body shape

It is beneficial to avoid a narrow exercise program where you only include running or another type of cardiovascular exercise. For optimal body composition, this is not ideal due to the catabolic effect of cardiovascular exercise. This simply means doing cardio work alone burns muscle as well as fat, so your overall body composition will be out of balance and you will not gain the tone and shape you desire. Remember, having **muscles give a toned look and great shape!** The added bonus is that **muscle helps burn fat!** Furthermore, if you follow a limited exercise program including only cardiovascular exercise, you will suppress the body's production of testosterone, which is needed for everyday function.

During a workout, aerobic exercise may burn more calories than weight training, yet weight training builds more lean muscle mass. These muscles then continue to burn calories even when your body is at rest. Increasing your lean muscle mass therefore increases your body's ability to burn calories both during and after your workout. Clearly, it is best to include both types of exercise in your program. Include exercises that target both your upper and lower body, choosing a weight that allows you to perform one set of 10 to 15 repetitions of each exercise. Aim to do some strength training two or more times per week. It does not necessarily have to be a separate session. I find it works best when I incorporate weight bearing exercise within an aerobic or anaerobic session. Aim to increase the number of sets and the weight you lift as your strength improves.

#2 Include aerobic AND anaerobic exercise in your program

Aerobic exercise is low intensity exercise where you maintain the same pace or intensity for a prolonged period of time. Examples include running, swimming, walking, and cycling, to mention just a few. The benefits of aerobic exercise are numerous, but in particular strengthening your heart and lungs. Anaerobic exercise is where the intensity of the exercise is too high to maintain for a long period of time, thus leading you take moments of rest between work 'intervals'. Typically you would work at a high intensity for 30-60 seconds with a 30-60 second break between these intervals, although these parameters can be varied. High intensity intervals can be performed running, rowing, swimming, cycling, with bodyweight exercises (circuits) or with weights. Like aerobic training, this form of training also works your heart and lungs well too. For example if you do a 10 minute warm-up, 6 sets of 30 seconds of work and 30 seconds of rest, rest for 2 minutes and do 3-4 blocks of this, each with a 2 minute rest period between, followed by a 10 minute cool down, your heart rate has been elevated for 50 minutes and your lungs will have had a great work out! This type of training is best for moms trying to lose baby weight ... the major benefit of anaerobic training being rapid and effective weight loss! Scientific research has revealed this to be **the best** form of weight loss training. Anaerobic training is even more effective if the interval training involves resistance provided by weights, medicine balls, sand bags or other types of implements, as opposed to performing intervals without resistance, for example running or cycling.

Sports such as soccer, hockey, netball and so on, contain both aerobic and anaerobic elements, and therefore are a great way to exercise and lose weight.

Bodyweight circuits, body pump and other similar exercise classes are good examples of aerobic sessions, which contain elements of anaerobic work interspersed throughout too. However, contrary to the understanding of many, you do not always need a gym or leisure center to provide exercise like this. With a little creativity and imagination it is possible to set your own sessions up at home or in the garden! Believe me, I meet a friend once week and we enjoy a great work out in the garden together. We get the music on, get some basic pieces of equipment ready, and hope that the sun shines!

Aerobic exercise burns calories, helps you regain some basic muscle strength and builds stamina. Start slowly with low-impact, calorie-burning exercises such as swimming, cycling, walking and the X-trainer. Experts recommend at least

30 minutes of physical activity five or more days a week for everyone. Obviously, as a new mom, you need to work towards this (more on progression later). It is quite easy for new moms to get plenty aerobic exercise. Simply taking your baby out in the pushchair for a daily brisk walk is perfect! Following an aerobics or dance DVD at home or attending a group fitness class for an effective aerobic workout will add variety. Build duration and intensity to your workouts as your strength and stamina improve.

#3 Exercise that improves function / General Conditioning

There are many exercises that can be done which have a positive impact on balance, stability, and body function. These exercises are sometimes done in exercise classes and can also be found on exercise DVD's. They work through fundamental movements that the body should be able to do, challenging balance and coordination. Examples of these types of exercises include lunges, squats, single leg squats, core exercises, overhead squats and arabesques. They give the body a level of robustness that lays a foundation for more rigorous forms of exercise, including weight training and high intensity intervals. These exercises also provide a strong base of conditioning for many popular activities such as sailing, canoeing, skiing, rock climbing and for participating in competitive sports such as netball, hockey, soccer, volleyball or dance. They strengthen the muscles, tendons, ligaments, connective tissue, and stabilize the joints. As a result, risk of injury is reduced.

#4 Exercise that improves Posture & Flexibility

If the types of exercises mentioned above are performed in a technically correct manner they provide two additional benefits. Firstly, they improve posture, allowing you to stand up straight and be well aligned from the tip of your head to the soles of your feet. This is important for long term health and mobility and can help to eradicate back pain or other forms of chronic pain. Evidently, good posture makes you look better and feel more confident. It even communicates a sense of confidence to others, which can be useful!

Secondly, if these exercises are performed through a full range of motion, as they should be, they will help to improve your joint mobility and flexibility. Joint mobility, along with good posture, unfortunately naturally decline with age, and therefore working on both of these areas becomes even more important. Many breastfeeding moms find they round their shoulders a lot whilst breastfeeding. This can lead to neck and shoulder pain and improper posture. Therefore, try to be aware of your posture during feeding. Find a comfortable and supported position where you do not have to hunch forward!

#5 General activity

Physical activity is important for health and longevity. Consequently it is important to be involved in a wide range of activities to strengthen different muscle groups and different aspects of fitness. As you include the fundamental principles of exercise explained in this chapter, it doesn't really matter what else you do, as long as you remain active. Being active plays a huge role in overall fitness and calories burned and for that reason it is good to make sure you are active in as many areas of your life as possible. Avoid living a sedentary life surrounding the exceptional moments when you drag yourself out for a jog, or go to your local leisure center to do an aerobics class. You need to be active throughout the day. When possible and realistic try walking rather than taking the car, take the stairs instead of the escalator, sit less and stand more, and play with your children in the park instead of sitting on a bench watching them play. I know some of my most precious memories with my boys are times we played in the park *together*. We have played countless games of catch, off-ground-tag, hide-and-seek, ball-tag, stuck-in-the-mud, soccer, fun races and many other active games (yes, I am the game playing queen!) Time flies by while you and your young children are having fun (and exercising!) Be creative in your games and be as active as you can!

Principles of exercise

One of the most commonly asked questions is "how soon after the baby is born can I start exercising?" To answer this question, it really depends on how long it takes for you to heal and *feel* ready to exercise again. Usually, it is 5 to 6 weeks before you feel like doing any intense exercise. And this, ideally, should be only done following a medical check. However, there are gentle exercises you can do from day one! I want to highlight the importance of doing pelvic floor exercises. I know many women skip these, not understanding the importance of them. I guess most people think that these exercises make no difference to their appearance or to the way they feel and therefore lack the motivation to do them. To explain, the pelvic floor muscles get weaker as you get older and especially following pregnancy. Weakened, they can cause problems including urinary incontinence and reduced sensitivity during sex. This is a new chapter of your life, so take this opportunity to start afresh. Be positive, be in control, and value yourself and your future. This is the very beginning of the new you. View these exercises as the first steps of your life journey with exercise being part of your lifestyle. You can't actually do much more on the first few days anyway, so please, just do them. By performing them you begin the reactivation of your core muscles, upon which, you will build. Let's be honest, it may be boring, but surely right now the thrill of having a new baby will get you through these dull moments of the day! You will notice improvement quickly, and believe me, the stronger they are the better for your future involvement in activities that involve any running or dancing or jumping! As a keen netball player (which requires lots of jumping and stretching) I experienced the concern of weakened pelvic floor muscles and so I worked on them!!! As you recover from labor and later down the line, you can do the star jump test to see if you need to continue to work on them!

I would encourage you to start going for short walks as soon as you feel able to do i.e. in the first week after birth. A little bit of fresh air everyday is good for you both physically and mentally. A short walk should leave you feeling refreshed and energized, and not exhausted. You can start with just a five-minute walk and build on this over time. Some moms manage to accumulate hours of walking in a day, especially when the baby sleeps well with the motion of the pushchair! Simply walking creates an excellent base level of fitness. As your fitness improves you will be able to extend the amount of time you walk and increase the pace.

In these first few weeks, your focus of exercise should not be weight loss, but merely getting out and about, being mobile, getting fresh air, catching up with friends and for your body to begin to feel normal again. If you are breastfeeding, you will certainly need energy to establish a good milk supply and therefore intense exercise at this point is not advisable. Even in the first few weeks many women notice some early weight loss. Some of this weight loss is due to the body getting rid of extra fluid gained during pregnancy, but some will also be fat loss. Experts suggest that a woman's body is designed to loose weight in the first 30 days following birth. Breastfeeding moms are often most aware of this initial weight loss. This is normal and natural so enjoy it.

The initial 5-6 weeks after having your baby is arguably the most exhausting. There are constant demands upon you and it is a time of great change and transition from life before motherhood to life now. Once you have recovered from this initial busy period, you will begin to feel that you have reached a greater physical and mental capacity and begin to desire more structured exercise. Some breastfeeding women find that they are no longer losing weight after the first 6-8 weeks. This is because the body has stabilized and got used to the excess calories that are being burned through feeding. Your body adapts and matches this demand by increasing calorie intake, thus negating the positive impact of breastfeeding for weight loss, and either stalling weight loss or even creating weight gain. If this has happened, or is happening to you, then it's a good time to reduce your calorie intake and start to exercise on a regular basis. Both these things will aid you in beginning to lose weight again.

Enjoy what you do!

As I have already said, I have met many people who aren't training for any particular event, yet they only partake in one form of exercise such as running or swimming. Some people even persevere with this one type of exercise despite the fact that they don't even enjoy it. I want to encourage you to try new things and to partake in a wide range of sports, classes, and activities. This keeps exercise fresh, challenging and rewarding as you continue to learn new skills, experience new places and meet new people. It helps avoid any possibility of boredom, which may lead to eventually quitting. I am not against choosing a sport or activity and sticking to it. There are benefits to this too. You see great improvement, you learn perseverance, and you achieve a much higher level in the chosen activity, experiencing great satisfaction! I am, however, trying to encourage those who are disillusioned with physical activity, those who seem to do the same old boring exercise, to try something new. I am sure everyone can find an activity that personally suits them and which they enjoy. Vary your activities, after all "variety is the spice of life". If you enjoy what you do, you are more likely to do it regularly and stick at it long enough to reap the benefits. If you enjoy exercising with others, do that. If you enjoy working out alone, do that. Discover your preference for being indoors or outdoors, being somewhere with music and noise or somewhere peaceful and tranquil. Find out what you enjoy and do it!

Make it feasible!

At this moment in time I am not a member of a gym and I cannot see this changing in the near future. The nearest gym is too far from home to make it practical for me to go to. My husband is away a lot with work and so most of the responsibilities of looking after the children are on me. My life is pretty full, most likely similar to yours. I simply don't have the time to make regular trips to the gym. In the past it has been different, but for now I am gym-less. But do not worry. Having no access to a gym does not mean I cannot exercise.

I have the privilege of living in a part of the world where the weather is great. I am able to play tennis outdoors for much of the year and ski for 4 to 5 months of the winter. On top of this, I enjoy going on walks and bike rides. I roller blade alongside the lake and occasionally go jogging. One evening a week I go to a Zumba class held in the village hall. At the age my boys are, it makes sense for me to choose primarily daytime outdoor activities that we can do together like cycling, swimming, and skiing. We do as much of these activities as possible. They enjoy them even more than I do!

In addition to this I lift weights at home (or in the garden) on a regular basis, either with my husband or with a friend, or I follow an exercise DVD. This helps me maintain some muscle to ensure that I keep the right body composition to stay in good shape, as mentioned earlier. I actually really enjoy weight training and find it leaves me feeling amazingly relaxed afterwards.

The message I want to communicate is both enjoyment and feasibility. Do not plan and strive for something that is simply not possible in the long term or stressful to organize as this will take away from the enjoyment. Do not try to maintain exercise routines which add stress instead of being de-stressing. If you have to drive an hour each way to the gym, then it's probably not a good idea to go to the gym. You need to find another form of exercise that fits easily in to your new rhythm of life. Remember you are not a mom to young children for a long time, so use this to motivate you in to new things. ...

It is great to be able to involve your baby for some of your fitness sessions thus negating the need to wait until the baby is asleep or the babysitter arrives before you get a decent workout. Put your baby in a sling or in the pushchair and get out for an interval power walking session, even pausing to do some lunges, press-ups or sit-ups if you are in a suitable environment such as a park or in the countryside. You could enroll in a moms and babies class where you exercise with your baby. The amount of exercises you can do whilst holding or being next to your child is amazing! Sit up peek-a-boo, squats with a baby carrier, bicep curls holing your baby, press-ups with baby lying on the floor under you, lunges holding your baby (I know one incredible mom of twins who did these with her girls, one in each arm!)

If you can get friends or family to look after your baby whilst you exercise, then that's great. Time without baby can be a welcomed relief! It can bring much needed time out from routine and responsibility, bringing a sense of freedom and relaxation. Sometimes it provides opportunity to simply focus on something/someone different and opportunity to re-focus on what is important. Sometimes motherhood becomes so busy we don't have time to think and reflect on our lives. Time out can help regain perspective in the difficult situations you may be facing or simply cause you to count your blessings!

Joining with other moms, with or without your babies, and doing some activity together is another great idea. Joining with others who are at similar stages in life can be so reassuring.

Essentially, you must be able to afford the time, support and the money to do the training or exercise that you choose. Again, at times you may need to be creative and think outside the box! Life with a newborn baby is not life as you have known it.

Progress, but progress slowly!

Please do not do the same session week in, week out without any change or progression. You will not be gaining the benefits you should be and you will soon become bored.

There is a principle in the science of training called "progressive overload" which was developed by Thomas Delorme, M.D. while he rehabilitated soldiers after World War II. He states that progressive overload is the gradual increase of stress placed upon the body during exercise training. Basically, in order to achieve more strength as opposed to maintaining the current strength capacity, the body's muscles must be overloaded. This overload stimulates the body's natural, adaptive processes to cope with the new demands placed on it. The adapted body is thus stronger than before the load had been placed on it.

I am a great believer in progressions. Once you have mastered one level in an exercise, and it begins to feel easier, your body has adapted and the muscles, tendons, ligaments and connective tissues are stronger, and you're ready to progress and move on to the next level. If there is no progression, there is no adaptation. Individuals who exercise sporadically never achieve any adaptation. They get the pains and aches after the initial session and then leave it so long before the next session that they never build on this. That means that whenever they return to exercise they are always at the same level. They never lift any heavier, run any faster or ride any further.

Always start easy, and progress. Once you have successfully completed the first exercises, pain free and with good technique you are ready to move on to the next level, and not before. Pushing yourself too hard too soon could cause injury, discouragement and breakdown.

Training can be progressed by increasing the pace, increasing the number of repetitions, increasing the number of sets, increasing the length of session, increasing the size off weights, changing the route you run. ... Note, you do not need to change all these factors at the same time. Choose one or two areas to change and progress slowly. Not only does this allow the body to adapt to new challenges, it helps overcome plateaus in form, and is definitely an antidote to boredom. I get bored quite easily; so progressing my sessions through making some changes mentioned above, keeps me interested and allows me to get fitter.

Free weights or weights machines?

Unless you have had an injury and are specifically carrying out rehab on a muscle or joint, you should stay away from weights machines and should lift dumbbells, kettle bells, barbells, sand bags or medicine balls. Machines work within a fixed plane of movement, making them excellent for early stages of rehab, and special situations, however for day-to-day training they are limited. The problem with machines is that they control the movement so that the body does not develop strength in multiple planes. This means that such movements do not prepare the body for real life situations. The muscles do not learn to balance and control the weights. In real life the body is required to absorb forces, control external loads and react to unpredictable movements. When the body is not prepared for this, it can end in injury. Training with free weights and the types of implements listed above allows your body to develop this strength, balance, control, and coordination. The ability to receive accurate perceptual information about joint position and movement, and respond to this is called proprioception. Lifting with free weights trains your *proprioception* as well as your *strength* and so is much more realistic to real life.

Consistency

This is probably the number 1 rule for exercise. It very much reinforces my philosophy of a lifetime of fitness. Fitness is not about the occasional workout or an active day here and there, and it's certainly not some distant memory in the past! It is a lifestyle choice. A commitment to health and well-being that is fun and enjoyable. Thus, when it comes to getting fit, lots of little sessions on a regular basis over a period of weeks, months, and years are much more effective than a really hard session every now and then. That doesn't mean I am not a believer of hard work. Of course it's good to push yourself, look for improvements and allow your body to adapt and get stronger and fitter. But it's good to remember that if you don't have the time for a long session, it's better to do something short than nothing at all. So many people think that since they don't have much time, they will wait and do a session when they have more time. This might be 3 or 4 days or even a week later. In that time they could have done 4 or 5 short, intense 15 minute sessions which is much more effective than one long 1 or even 2 hour session! So remember "Little and Often". A few lunges and squats can take just a few minutes!

Spot reduction is impossible!

The term spot reduction is used to suggest you can choose an area of your body and target that area for specific fat reduction. This is impossible. There is a lot of misinformation out there. There are people selling machines, which they claim to burn fat on your bum or your thighs or your tummy. ... The truth is, that none of these work. Let's have a look at why.

If someone wants to lose fat on their stomach

and they do lots of abdominal exercises, yes, their abs will get stronger. However, there will be no noticeable difference from the outside. Their abs will remain covered in a thick layer of fat. The tone that people are striving for is simply not going to happen unless you loose fat throughout the whole of your body. If you want to shrink your midsection, you'll need to lose weight all over your body, accomplished through a sensible diet, low in refined sugar and processed foods. This, alongside strength training, combined with 30 minutes of daily aerobic activity will create the desired toned stomach. Isolating the abs and only working on these is not the best overall plan. My husband coaches many athletes whom do very little, if any, isolated abdominal work, and yet have the most amazing 6-packs ever!

The bottom line is simple. You need to decrease body fat through dietary manipulation and exercise. The combination of reduced body fat and increased lean muscle mass leads to a more "toned" look.

What about Energy levels?

Your ability to exercise is dependent on your energy levels and your psychological state i.e. how you feel about exercising. Many people believe that if they *feel* they don't have the energy to exercise then they should not exercise. However, your felt energy levels can be affected by the amount of sleep you have had, the mood you are in, what you have eaten, your blood sugar levels, your caffeine intake and your level of desire for exercise. If you consistently get too little sleep, have one sugar spike or caffeine spike after the next, chances are you are very rarely going to *feel* like you have the energy to exercise. Sitting on the sofa with another cup of coffee and a chocolate bar *seems* far more appealing and *feels* like what your body needs, when actually; exercise is most likely exactly what your body needs! Exercising can actually be extremely energizing, and missing out on your exercise session could make you feel like you have even less energy!

To get a 'fair' and true reflection of your actual energy levels there are several areas to consider. You need to make sure you are getting to bed early to ensure as much sleep as possible when you have a new baby to care for during the night. Being sleep deprived will have a negative impact on your ability to exercise. You should be eating a diet with fewer sugar spikes, and not drinking too much caffeine. Both these factors can impact your desire to exercise and quality of exercise session. Both can mask how you are actually feeling in a positive or negative way. A sugar spike and the following low can make you *feel* tired and lethargic when actually you have plenty glycogen energy stores in your muscles and you are capable of a great exercise session and are ready to go!

Sssssssssleep...

As you have read in my chapter titled Rest, Recovery and Sleep, sleep is extremely important in the post pregnancy period. Most people know that sleep is important for your health, but once you start adding exercise into your busy schedule, its importance increases.

It may be a difficult concept to understand but a good workout breaks down your body and it's the effective and adequate rest and sleep that follows that repairs it and makes it stronger. Therefore, no matter how hard you train, if you don't get sufficient sleep, you are compromising your recovery and subsequent training, and in effect wasting your time. The best results come when you work hard and rest well. During deep sleep, growth hormone production increases. It is this which helps to repair and rebuild muscles, and build strong bones after training. It is also worth noting that growth hormone production and release also promotes fat burning!

The National Sleep Foundation in the USA state that while naps cannot make up for inadequate night time sleep, a quick nap of 20-30 minutes may improve your mood, alertness and performance of tasks. Further research in a NASA study suggested that a 40-minute nap improved the performance of sleepy military pilots and astronauts by 34% and increased alertness by 100%. Therefore, I urge you to take a nap if the opportunity arises, especially if you have exercised. If it works for astronauts it works for moms!

Interestingly though, not only is sleep essential for rest and recovery, and for adaptation to exercise, but inversely, exercise is key to achieving good sleep. In fact, studies show that those struggling with insomnia should exercise more, and the more intense the exercise, the better the sleep that follows!

Exercise or Good Nutrition- Which is more important?

Exercise alone, is not the optimum source of weight loss. Exercise needs to be combined with a healthy eating plan in order to lose weight the best way. In fact, in some cases, people who exercise vigorously and regularly, yet have poor nutrition are unable to lose weight or achieve their desired body composition. On the other hand, there are individuals who look slim and fit, and perhaps have a good diet, however, they do not exercise, and therefore are not as healthy as they might look. Therefore whatever your motivation for exercise, whether for health or body shape, or something else, you should realize that your exercise must be combined with good nutrition! You should not exercise solely to lose weight; after all, once you've achieved your ideal weight you won't need to lose any more. Be motivated by the fact that you are improving your health for you and your family, which in turn will allow you to live your life to the full!

Tips before you start

- Keep in mind what your body has been through and don't expect too much too soon. Do not put yourself under unnecessary pressure to get fit overnight. Be realistic.

- Good breast support is necessary. You should make sure you get a good support bra as your breasts will be larger than normal and if you are breastfeeding they are also likely be tender. If you do not get the right support you may feel uncomfortable when you exercise.

- You only need the bare minimum in terms of equipment. A set of gym clothes, a comfortable pair of trainers and a floor mat will be sufficient.

During each exercise session start slowly and increase your intensity gradually but steadily. This also applies to your exercise routine as a whole.

Be aware that after pregnancy your ligaments may be lax, leading to hyper-mobility, particularly round the hip and pelvic areas. Therefore, for the first few months do not work to extreme ranges of motion to avoid putting unnecessary pressure on your joints.

Drink regularly during and after exercise particularly if you are breastfeeding. Your body requires water for many of its vital functions.

Getting started

Getting started is one of the hardest things. Not just because of the lack of motivation, but more so due to the fact that many people do not know what to do to actually get started! Below is an outline, showing a safe and effective process from recovering from birth, to gentile exercise, to high level training for weight loss and gaining a great post pregnancy body.

Although realistically, much of a mom's motivation to exercise is to regain previous body shape, exercise should be stress-relieving not stress-provoking. The American Council on Exercise suggests that the goal of exercise after giving birth should be to help with relaxation, stress management, rehabilitation and emotional well-being rather than the goal of getting your previous body back.

When you initially try to do any kind of stomach exercises, you will very quickly realize that you simply can't. Your abdominal muscles have been stretched and in most cases pulled apart and no longer work! Don't panic. You are able to quickly re-learn how to use them and re-train them to work effectively by following the step-by-step progression of exercises that follow. This is a time in your life when you will need to do a lot of abdominal work to recover their position, heal and re-gain their strength. Once you have gone through this process, you will be able to maintain a strong core by doing very little isolated abdominal work and concentrating more on whole body movements (which also work your abs).

You should not feel that you need to slow down after having a baby. Of course you will feel tired at times, especially during the first 4-6 weeks, that's normal, but you should be as active as you can be. Get plenty of rest when baby is sleeping and if you can, go to bed early. Remember, sleep helps heal the body and aids in recovery from exercise.

One of the biggest things on your mind is probably losing the weight you gained while you were pregnant. Remember that it took nine months to gain the weight, (which was distributed in a certain manner to support pregnancy and breastfeeding), and this weight gain did and does serve a purpose! Now, the process of losing this weight will take a similar amount of time. Be gentle with yourself, and give yourself the time to lose the weight in a healthy, positive way!

Post pregnancy return to exercise – The START of the program

Level 1 – Abdominal Breathing Exercises & Pelvic Floor Exercises

(Weeks 1-2)

The easiest way to get started with exercise is by doing Abdominal Breathing Exercises. These can be done as early as day 1. Although these exercises are not strenuous, the abdominal muscles can be strengthened through abdominal breathing, whilst the body relaxes. Lie flat on your back on the floor with your head supported by pillows. Gently place one hand on top of your abdomen and inhale deeply. As you inhale, the abdomen will rise higher. Hold this for five seconds, and then slowly release the air, watching the abdomen fall back to its original position. Hold this position for five seconds, repeating the process four to six times.

Pelvic floor exercises, called Kegel exercises after the gynecologist who created them, can and should be done within the first few days after birth. They require no gym membership, exercise mat or even a need to put aside time for this "exercise session". In fact they can be done standing up, sitting down watching TV, waiting for the bus, or anywhere really – and no one will know you're doing them! Kegel exercises don't just strengthen the pelvic floor, but they also help support the abdomen similarly to the abdominal breathing exercises.

If you wish to lie down, lie flat on your back and bend your knees with your feet flat on the floor. Relax your head on the floor and look up at the ceiling. Contract the muscles of your vagina as if you are trying to stop the flow of urine. Make sure you are not just contracting your bum muscles. Hold this for 4-5 seconds. Repeat 10 times. Do 3-5 sets of this spaced throughout the day.

It's important to first build your pelvic floor muscles and deep core muscles through doing these exercises before you begin to work on your superficial abdominal muscles. Skipping this step will slow your progress and cause slow adaptation to other core work.

The Level 1 exercises can be carried on throughout Level 2 and Level 3 for as long as you feel necessary. In fact, by doing these pelvic floor exercises for 6-8 weeks, you will get an added benefit.

Level 2 – Early Progressions of Core Exercises

(Weeks 2-4)

The core is an important part of the body that acts as a support to all movements that the human body makes. It is the center of control and from it the arms and legs operate. To me, the core consists of more than just the abdominal muscles. The core consists of the whole mid-section of the body, which includes the abdominals, hips, pelvis, and lower back. The core plays an essential role in posture, which is vital for overall health and vitality. Moreover, posture is important for being able to execute exercises correctly.

Initially after birth, there is a gap in the abdominals that will take time to knit back together. It feels odd and there is the sensation that you have no strength in your abs at all. You are likely to be unable to perform simple tasks. Even sitting up to get out of bed may be a challenge, and you may find yourself having to first roll onto your side in order to get out of bed. These specific exercises have been chosen because they will help to close the gap that was formed during pregnancy, regain the strength and function of your abs, and enable you to get back to normal. You will even be able to use these alongside other exercises and methods to get a flat stomach and even a 6 pack if that's what you want!

Checklist

- Make sure you perform each exercise with good form.
- It's better to start with 3-5 repetitions done well, than 10 repetitions done poorly
- Work up to 2-3 sets of 10 repetitions (except where otherwise stated)
- Work through the range of motion that your body allows you to and progress towards working through a full range of motion. (Warning – during the first 6 weeks after birth DO NOT push your ligaments to their maximum capacity – see earlier in chapter)
- Think about breathing in during the easy part of the movement and breathing out at the end of the effort.
- Remember "form, posture, breathing"

When you have mastered all of the core exercises in Level 2, move on to Level 3 but not before.

Seated isometric Abs squeezes
Try sitting up tall and squeezing your belly inwards to your spine. Start with 20 each day, working up to 100 each day.

Pelvic tilts
Stand straight with your back to the wall and relax your spine. Breathing in deeply, and press the small of your back against the wall. Exhale and repeat. Continue the exercise for 1-2

minutes. These can be repeated several times throughout the day.

Happy cat, angry cat

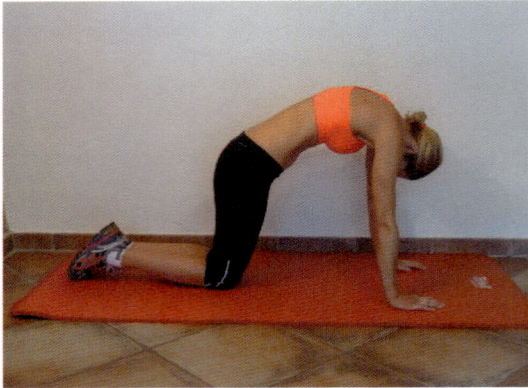

Kneel on all fours and round your back with your head pointing downwards. Tilt your pelvis forwards.

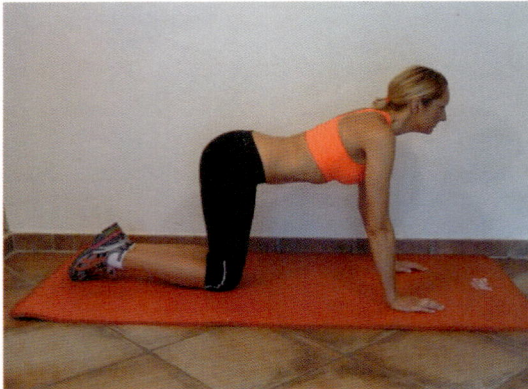

Slowly transition to an arched back position with your head looking upwards and your pelvis tilted backwards.

Single arm drop

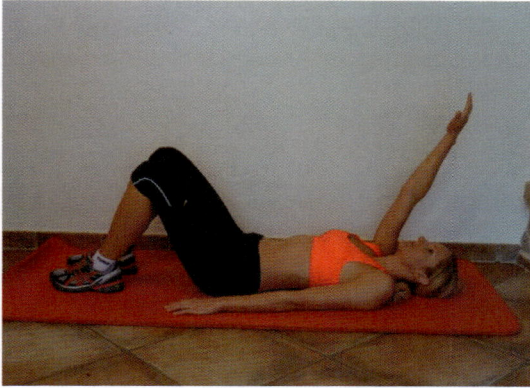

Lie flat on your back with your arms by your side, head looking upwards and spine neutral. Bend your knees and put your heels on the floor. Raise one arm upwards and above your head. Move your arm slowly backwards and forwards whilst maintaining your neutral spine position (there should be no movement in your back).

Single leg drop

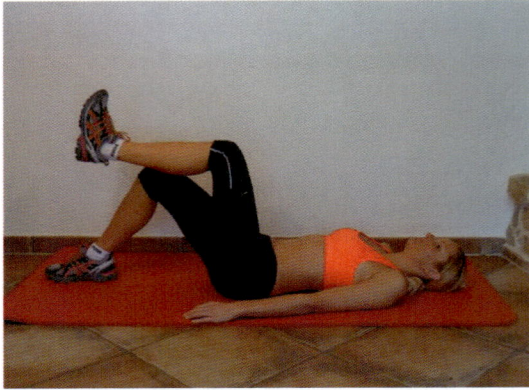

Lie flat on your back with your arms by your side, head looking upwards and spine neutral. Bend your knees and put your heels on the floor. Raise one knee upwards towards your chest, and then back to its resting position.

Double leg hip bridge

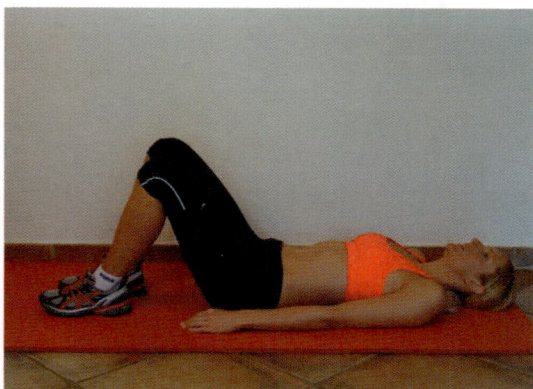

Lie flat on your back with your arms by your side, head looking upwards and spine neutral. Bend your knees and put your feet flat on the floor.

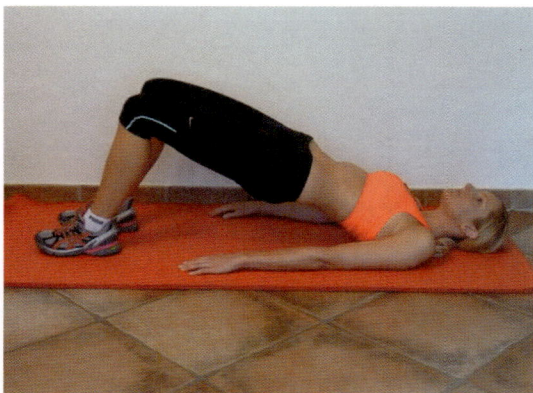

Pushing your feet into the floor and squeezing your glutes (buttocks), raise your hips upwards until you achieve a straight line from your knees to your shoulders. Return to the start position and repeat this.

Fire Hydrants

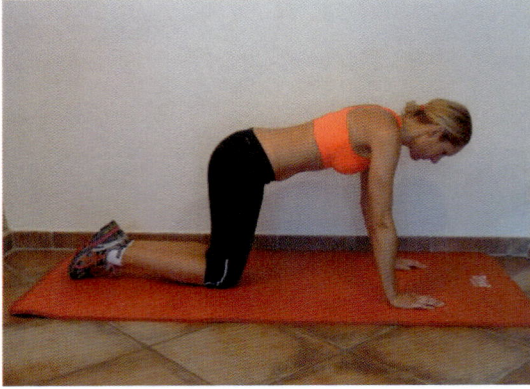

Kneel on all fours, and hold your tummy in whilst maintaining a flat back. Keep your head in a neutral position.

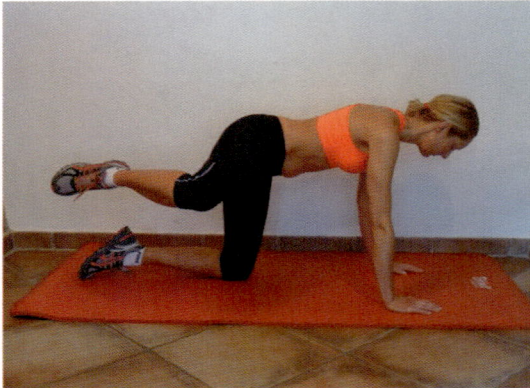

Slowly lift one leg out sideways and then back to the start position whilst maintaining a neutral spine and head position throughout.

4-point kneeling arm raise

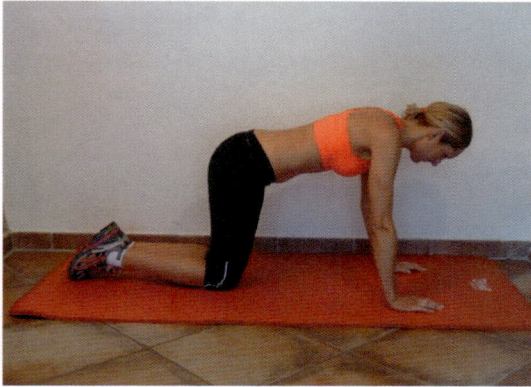

Kneel on all fours, and hold your tummy in whilst maintaining a flat back. Keep your head in a neutral position.

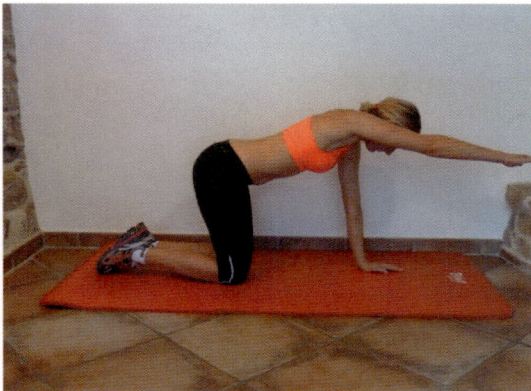

Slowly lift one arm out in front then place it back to the floor. Maintain a neutral spine and head position throughout.

4-point kneeling leg raise

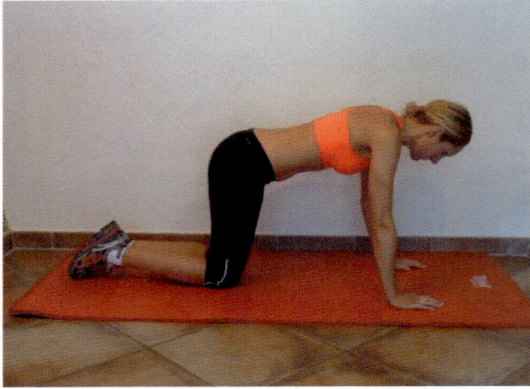

Kneel on all fours, and pull your tummy in, maintaining a flat back. Keep your head in a neutral position.

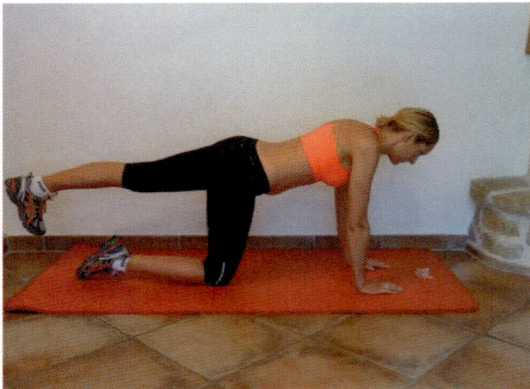

Slowly lift one leg out behind then place it back to the floor. Maintain a neutral spine and head position throughout.

Clams

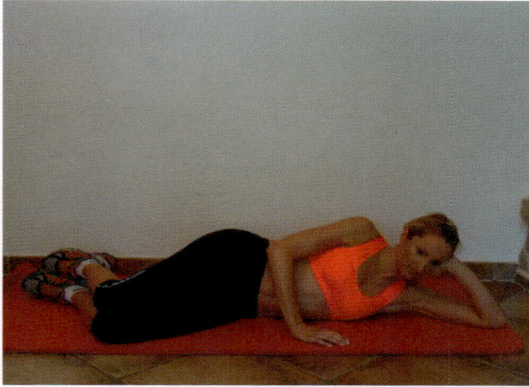

Lie on your side with your head supported in your hand and bend both legs comfortably underneath you.

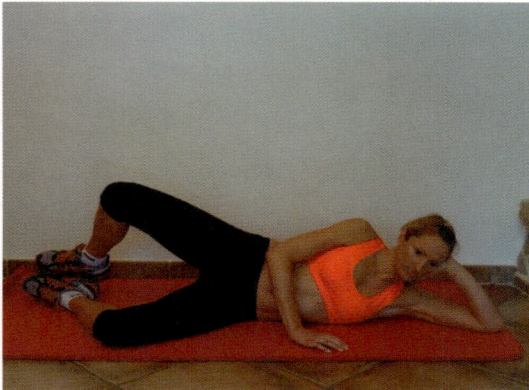

Slowly lift your knee upwards, initiating the movement from your glutes whilst keeping your hips in the same position.

Side lying knee lift

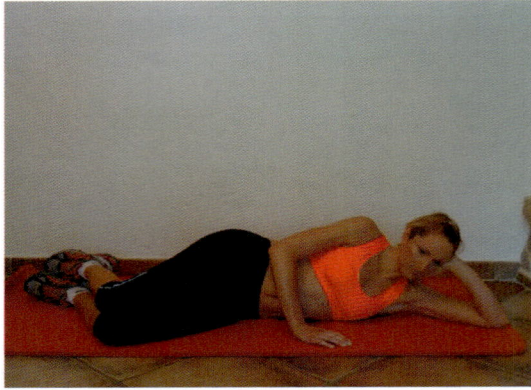

Lie on your side with your head supported in your hand and bend both legs comfortably underneath you.

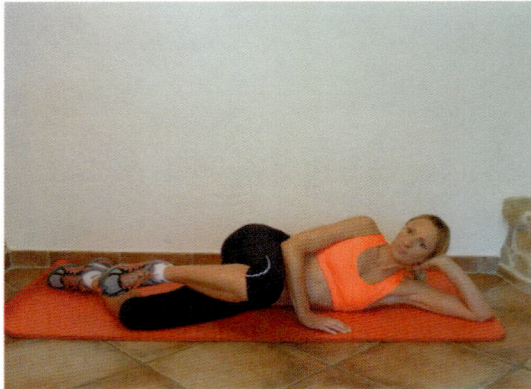

Bring the knee of your top leg upwards towards your chest then back to a straight position in line with your body.

Knee lift & kickbacks

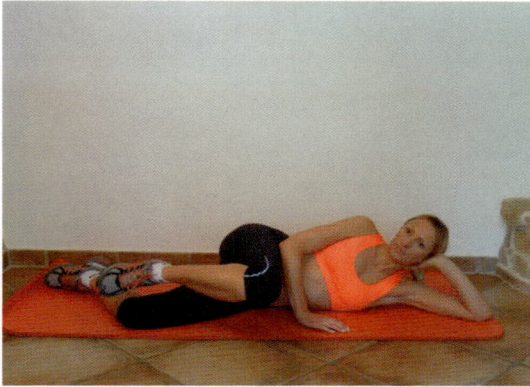

Lie on your side with your head supported in your hand and bend both legs comfortably underneath you. Bring the knee of your top leg upwards towards your chest.

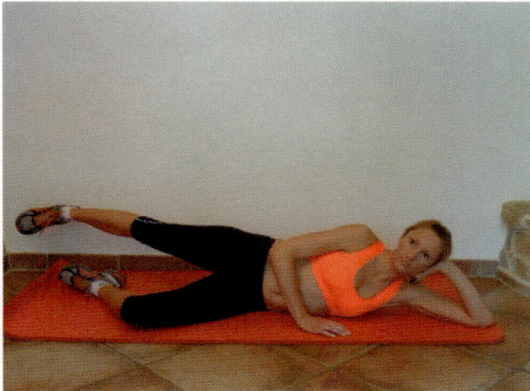

Extend the leg backwards and kick out behind you whilst maintaining your body posture.

Heel touch

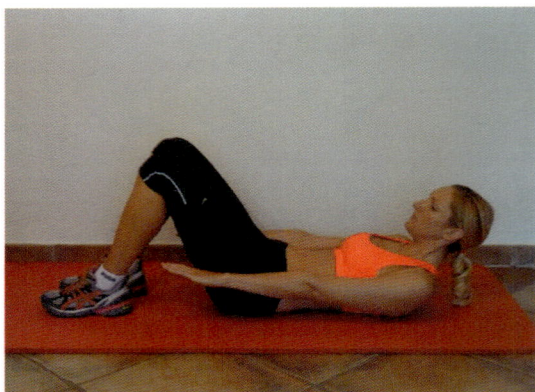

Lie on your back with your knees bent, heels flat on
the floor, and arms by your side. Crunch upwards,
slightly raising your shoulders off the mat.

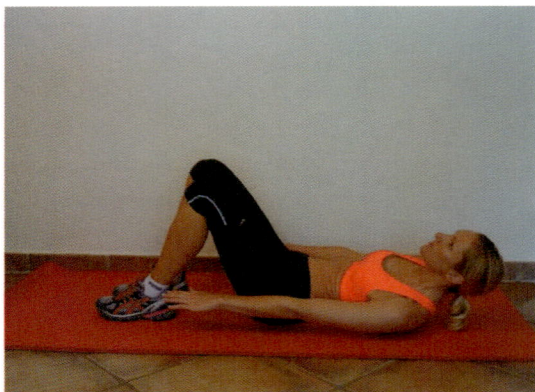

Move side-to-side moving your hand towards your
heel, without letting your shoulders touch the mat.

Single leg fallouts

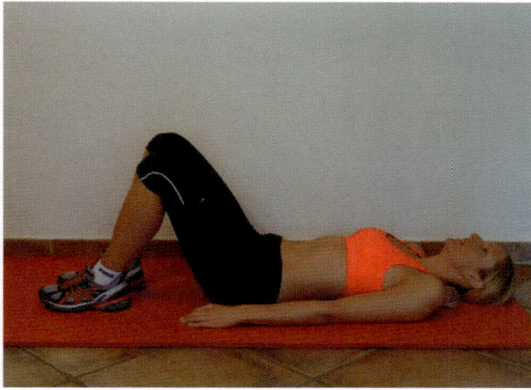

Lie flat on your back with your arms by your side.
Keep your head looking upwards and spine neutral.
Bend your knees and lift one foot off the floor binging
the knee towards the chest.

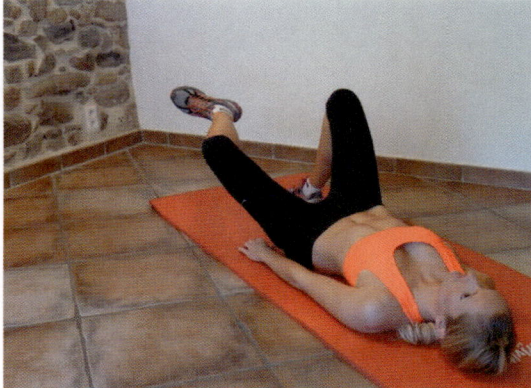

Allow the leg which is off the floor to fallout to one
side through movement of the hip joint, and then
bring this knee back to the start position.

Hip drops

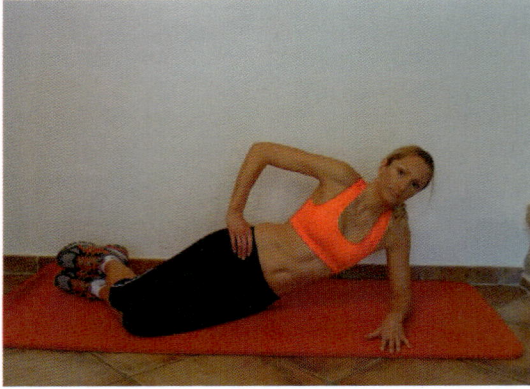

Lie on your side with your elbow and knees on the floor and one hand on your hip.

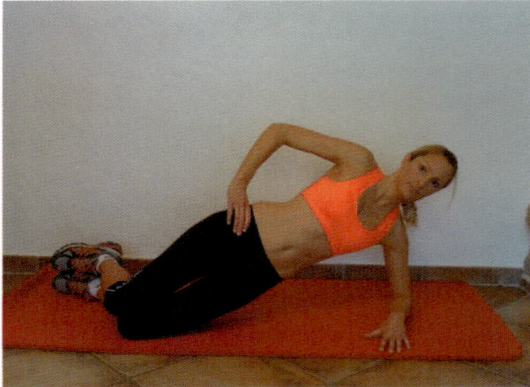

Lift your hips upwards to the position where your body is in a straight line and lower your hips down again. Do this repeatedly.

Half side plank

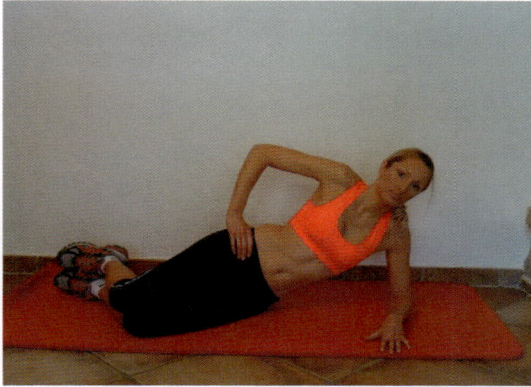

Lie on your side with your elbow and knees on the
floor and one hand on your hip.

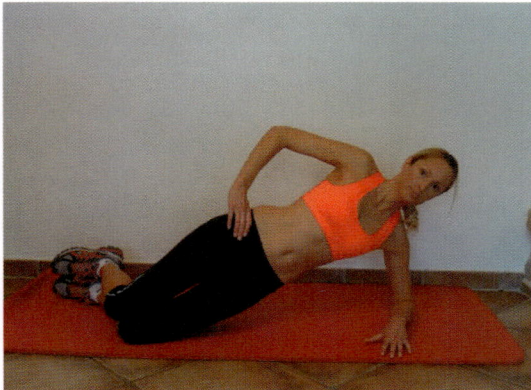

Lift your hips upwards to the position where your
body is in a straight line and hold this position until
you begin to lose form. Work up to 1 minute.

Level 3 – Further Progressions of Core Exercises

(Weeks 4-6)

The following exercises are progressions of the earlier exercises shown in Level 2. They are more difficult to perform. If you cannot perform Level 2 exercises correctly, you will not be able to perform the following ones with good form. As a result you will be putting your body at risk of injury. Only when you are able to perform 2-3 sets of 10+ repetitions of the Level 2 exercises with no pain and with perfect form, are you ready to move onto the further progressions of the core exercises.

The exercises in Level 3 follow the same principles as the ones above. Progress slowly from 3-5 repetitions until you can perform 2-3 sets of 10 repetitions (except where otherwise stated). Ensure good form for each repetition, in order not to put your body at risk of injury.

Double bent leg lift

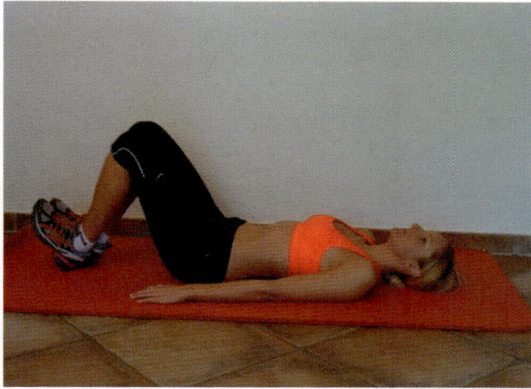

Lie flat on your back with your arms by your side, head looking upwards and spine neutral. Bend your knees and put your heels on the floor.

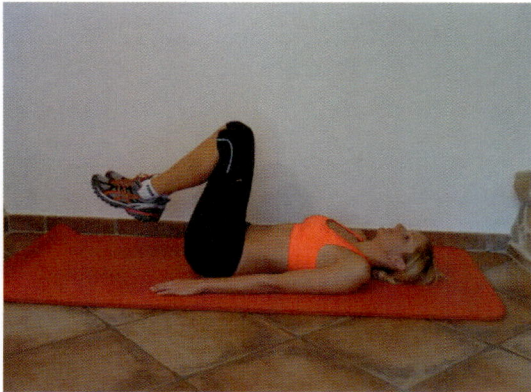

Slowly raise your knees upwards towards your chest whilst maintaining a flat back. Draw your abs in whilst maintaining relaxation throughout the rest of your body.

Single Straight leg lift

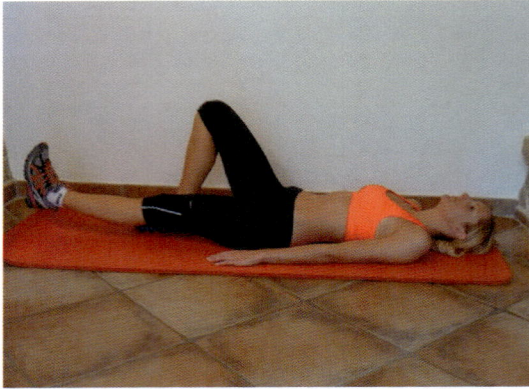

Lie flat on your back with your arms by your side, head looking upwards and spine neutral. Bend one leg and keep the other leg straight.

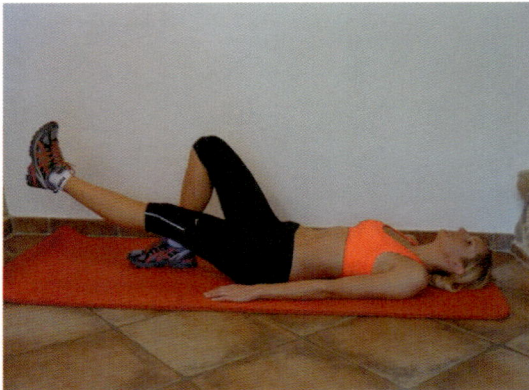

Slowly lift the straight leg off the floor. Initially use your hands to help by pushing into the floor. Progress this by turning your palms upwards and not using your hands to push. Maintain a neutral spine throughout the movement.

Leg bounces at 90°

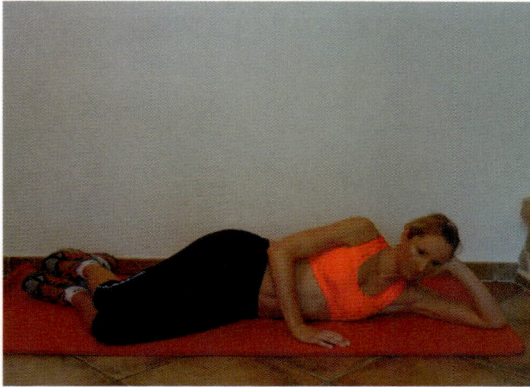

Lie on your side with your head supported in one hand and the other hand on the floor in front of you for support.

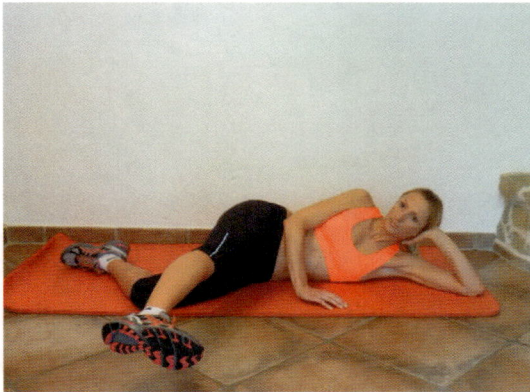

Extend your top leg out in front at 90° and bounce up and down with small movements for 30 seconds

Opposite Arm and leg lifts

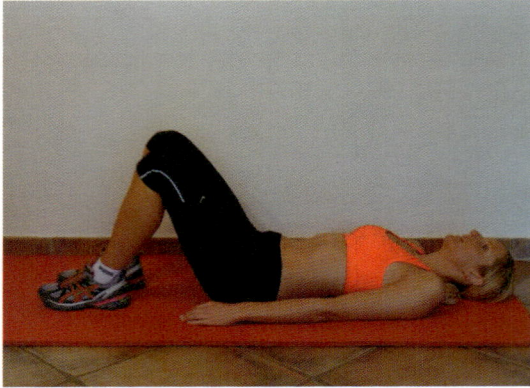

Lie flat on your back with your arms by your side, head looking upwards and spine neutral. Bend your knees and put your feet flat on the floor.

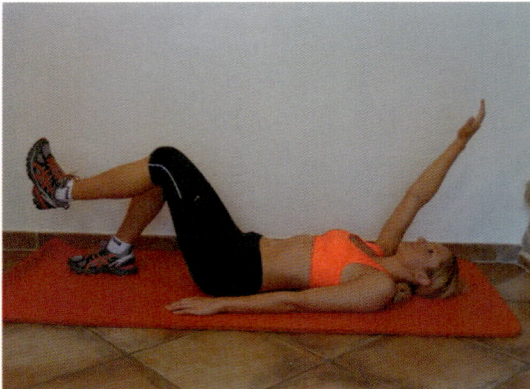

Lift one arm and the opposite leg. As you lower your leg, lower your arm. Repeat with the other arm and leg.

Dead bugs

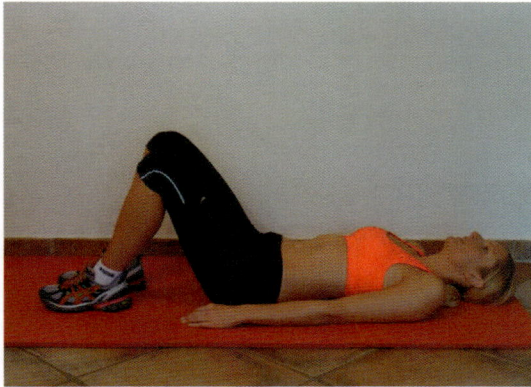

Lie flat on your back with your arms by your side, head looking upwards and spine neutral. Bend your knees and put your feet flat on the floor.

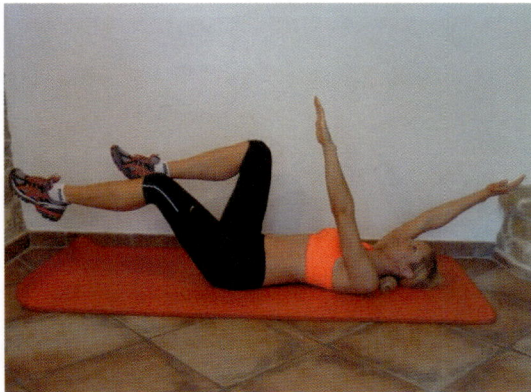

Lift one arm and the opposite leg. Stretch your arm above your head and lower the opposite leg to the floor simultaneously. Repeat with the other arm and leg so that both arms and legs are moving simultaneously in opposite directions.

Front plank

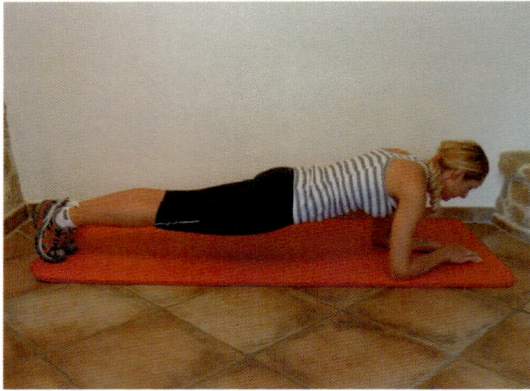

Hold your body as flat as possible with your weight on your forearms and toes. Maintain a straight line through your body with your head in a neutral position. Hold still for as long as you can until you lose form. Work up to 1 minute.

Crunch

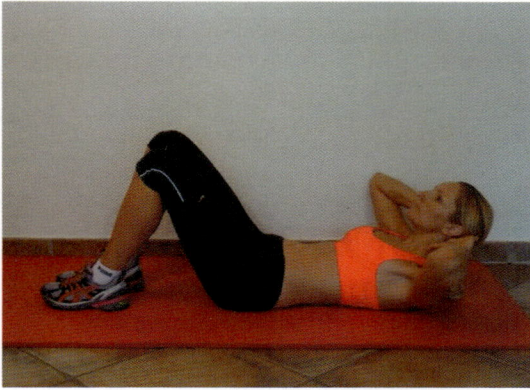

Lie flat on your back with your knees bent and feet flat on the floor. Place your hands behind your head for support. Slowly crunch upwards by raising your shoulders off the mat. Return slowly to the start position.

Single leg hip bridge

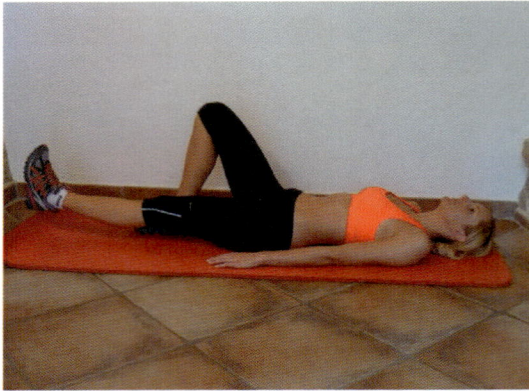

Lie flat on your back with your arms by your side, head looking upwards and spine neutral. Bend one knee and keep the other leg straight.

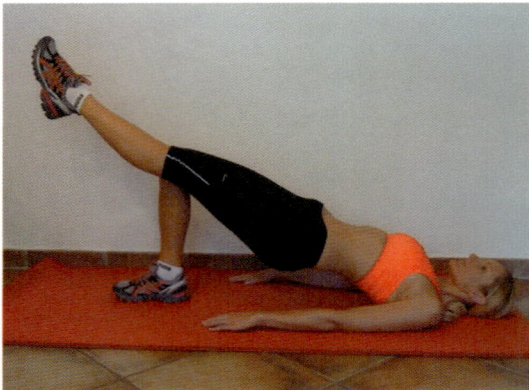

Pushing your foot into the floor and squeezing your glutes (buttocks), raise your hips and leg upwards until you achieve a straight line from the toe of your extended leg to your shoulders. Lower your hips back down to the mat to return to the start position. Work up to 10 repetitions. Repeat on the same number with the opposite leg.

4-point kneeling, opposite arm and leg raise

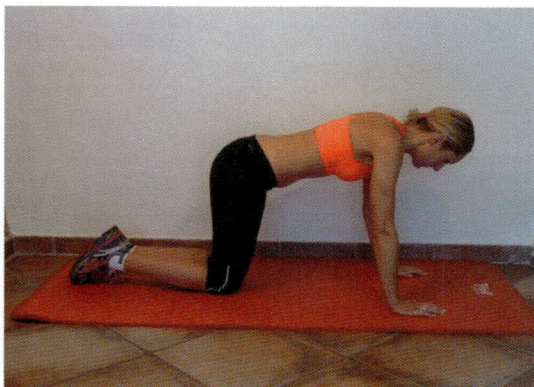

Kneel on all fours, hold your tummy in maintaining a flat back and keep your head in a neutral position.

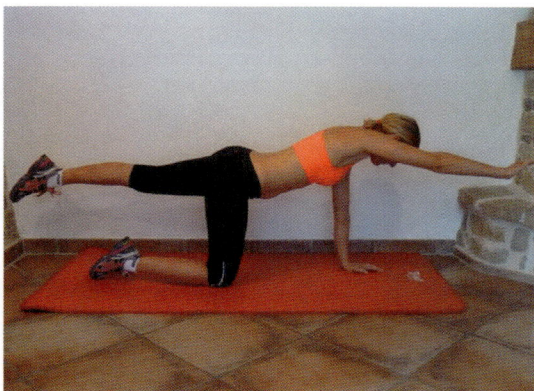

Slowly and simultaneously lift one arm out in front, and the opposite leg out behind then place them back to the floor. Repeat on the other side. Maintain a neutral spine and head position throughout the movement.

Half side plank with leg lift

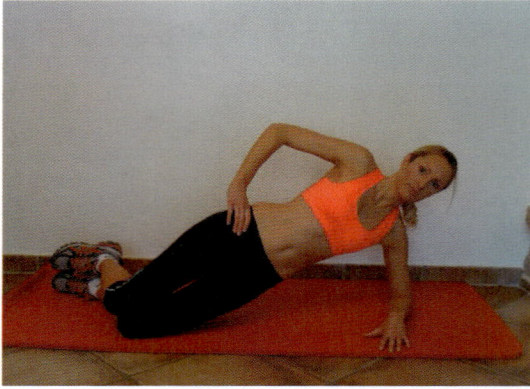

Hold the half side plank position described in Level 2, with your weight on your knees and forearm.

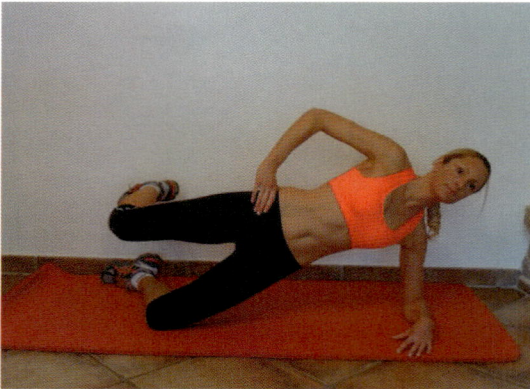

Either raise your knee up and down whilst maintaining a strong core, or raise your knee upwards and hold this position for as long as you can without losing form.

Side plank

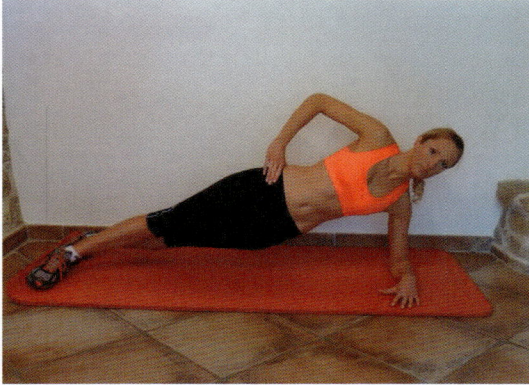

Lie on your side then raise your weight off the mat so that all your weight rests on your forearm and feet. For balance, place the foot of your top leg in front of the foot of your back leg.

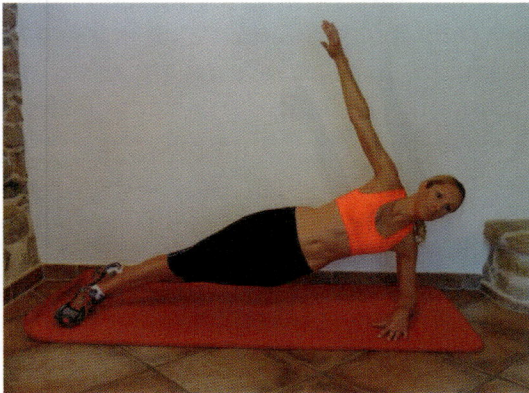

Vary this by either raising your hand into the air, or by raising one leg up like in the half side plank above.

During week 4-6, whilst you are doing Level 3, you should aim to swim or walk regularly in addition to performing the core exercises. Both swimming and walking provide muscle toning, low impact workouts. The heart and lungs benefit too. Swimming, however, may have to wait until you stop secreting lochia. As soon as the discharge finishes, you're ready to go.

Level 4 – Full-body Conditioning, Jogging, & Cycling

(Weeks 6-10)

As you progress through the first 3 levels and can feel your body getting stronger and fitter, you are ready to continue further to full-body conditioning exercises, jogging and cycling. As you begin to increase the intensity and duration, you can begin to play some sport again or take part in more rigorous exercise. I have encouraged waiting until this point to start sport or vigorous forms of exercise again. This is due to the fact that until now, your ligaments have been lax and your body has not been used to the extreme range of movements and the speed of these movements, and so could easily get injured. Rebuilding a strong base first means that you are more likely to stay injury free and enjoy training problem free.

The overall plan at this point is to get into full body workouts and other activities such as sports, aerobic classes, or strength programs. These exercises in your workouts should be based round functional movements that apply to daily life.

Lifting weights will improve your strength and functional ability to perform daily tasks. Performed with correct technique it also protects your joints and can reduce back pain. I therefore like to recommend some form of weight training.

Progress from core/floor work to full body conditioning! Here are some excellent exercises that I like to include at different times in a training program:

- Push-ups with knees on the floor or push-ups with feet on the floor
- Other pushing exercises like bench press and push press (varying between bar and dumbbells)
- Pull-ups with bands to aid
- Other pulling exercises like horizontal pulls to a bar and bent over row
- Squatting, including wide sumo style squats and single leg squats
- Overhead squats (bar above the head)
- Step-ups (onto a bench or step with dumbbells or a barbell)
- Lunges (forwards and backwards)
- Lateral lunges
- Arabesque (Single leg "good morning" or Single leg Romanian dead lift)

Romanian dead lift

These exercises should first be mastered using your body weight and being performed for 3 sets of 10-12 repetitions without loss of form. Once this can be done well, you can add weight to these and see yourself progress. If these exercises are new to you and you want to use weights, I recommend learning them under the supervision of a Personal Trainer or Coach. Otherwise you may not be doing them correctly and could be putting yourself at risk of injury.

Level 5 – Strength Training & all forms of Sport

(Weeks 8-12 and onwards) Yippee!!!

Once you reach this stage you have laid an excellent foundation through progressing your exercises and abilities over an 8 to 10 week period. You are now ready to progress to higher intensity exercises or exercise classes, weight training, interval training or sports.

There are so many different sports and activities that you can enjoy to keep fit. I'm hoping that through your journey back to fitness after having your baby, or perhaps your journey to fitness for the first time, you have felt inspired to try something different. This could be buying a new exercise DVD that involves exercises that you have never done before. It could be taking up a new sport, or joining a new club or class. You may decide to take up CrossFit, or train for a 5K race, a triathlon, or maybe a half marathon or even marathon! You may, like me, chose to do a mixture of activities. I enjoy weight training, exercise DVDs, circuit-style training, Zumba, skiing, roller blading, cycling, swimming, tennis and occasional jogging (!). The opportunities are vast.

You may have met new people or made new friends through attending exercise classes, or through going to the gym. Whatever has changed for you going through this process, I want to encourage you to stay active, fit and healthy.

Stretching

Stretching is an important form of exercise, especially after a workout. If you spend a small amount of time stretching each major muscle group that you have used in the exercise session, it will help your recovery. Stretching relaxes the muscles and helps realign the muscle fibers, causing them to return to their pre-exercise state. If you find it hard to stretch regularly, or don't really know the best way to do it, you may benefit from a Yoga class, as this is a great way of stretching. Stretching is also good for maintaining and improving flexibility, which is an important aspect of health and fitness. As we age, we lose flexibility in our muscles and joints, and therefore are at greater risk of injury. By maintaining, or improving flexibility, we are reducing our risk of injury and extending our functional physical ability i.e. our ability to perform daily tasks.

Resuming exercise after a C-section

A caesarean section, also called a C-section, is major abdominal surgery that involves a surgical incision through the uterus and abdomen. It is therefore necessary to acknowledge that it will inevitably take longer to recover from, than a virginal birth. A full recovery comes over a matter of months, not days, and can sometimes be difficult. Normal, everyday tasks and situations you once took for granted can become a challenge. For example the simple task of getting out of bed with ease and pleasure, driving, or wearing your favorite jeans can all be affected by the surgery.

Although you may be eager to return to your pre-pregnancy shape after a C-section, it is important to allow yourself plenty of time to heal and recover before returning to an exercise plan. Most obstetricians recommend a recovery period of at least six to eight weeks before engaging in vigorous exercise like sit-ups, interval training, weight training or playing sports. There are however, plenty of things you *can* do in this initial period. I believe waiting 6 weeks and then suddenly doing something really physically tough is not a good idea. Dramatically changing your level of engagement in physical activity is dangerous. Moving from no participation in exercise to blasting out a demanding exercise session can cause injury and halter recovery. Equally damaging is the mental consequence of this behavior. You are likely to find it extremely difficult and discouraging and are likely to feel sore afterwards. The combination of these factors are likely to put you off exercising in the future. Consequently, during this initial six week period, instead of simply waiting, you can engage in very gentle, foundational work. Start with some low level exercises and progress slowly, just like anyone recovering from a natural birth. Keep in mind that you need to start gently and progress slowly, little by little. You are recovering from both minor surgery and 9 months of pregnancy!

The process of recovery is slightly different from that of a virginal birth and there are a number of important factors to consider. No doubt your health visitor will guide you in some aspects of recovery. I believe, however, it is of paramount importance to outline certain key points.

You simply cannot avoid all exercise and then suddenly begin to exercise like you used to in your times of peek fitness. Progression is vital! Returning to exercise should look something like this:

Day 1

You will be in hospital and will be well looked after. Other than for feeding baby, you should use this time for bed rest, sleep and relaxation. If you need to get up you should always get help from a nurse and not cause yourself any unnecessary pain by trying to get up alone. Do not get up from your bed for the first time without help from a nurse.

Day 2

Within the first 24 hours, you may want to get out of bed and do some slow walking in your room or down the hospital corridor. Moving around really is important for your recovery. Range-of-motion exercises in bed or even some light walking should be done as soon as possible after your C-section to help minimize muscle wasting and increase circulation which promotes healing. Examples of exercises to get the blood going in your legs include wiggling your feet, rotating your ankles, and moving and stretching your legs slowly as you lie in bed. Try to take your walks a short time after you've taken your pain medication, when you're likely to feel more comfortable. You can start doing abdominal breathing exercises mentioned earlier on in this chapter. Regulate these by the amount of pain you feel. There is no reason to inflict any pain on yourself – you should be totally pain free whilst performing them. If you feel you are unable, please don't panic. Leaving it another day or so is not going to harm you. The reason I recommend getting started on day 2 is that many moms find it easier psychologically to do something early on.

Day 3-5

Depending on which country you live in and the system of care there, you will generally be allowed to go home 3 to 5 days after delivery. Whilst you are still in hospital, take advantage of the help that you can get. If you are in hospital you should continue with small amounts of walking down the corridors, and stretching in bed. Continue with the abdominal breathing exercises and introduce Kegal exercises whilst lying in bed. If you go home during this time, make sure you have sufficient help so that you do not have to do any physical tasks around the house. If possible even avoid bending and lifting the baby. Getting others to pass baby to you is best.

If you can, avoid walking upstairs in the first few days that you're at home. If not, walk up the stairs backwards as it can help minimize the chance of using your abdominal muscles to stand up straight as you extend your leg.

You will probably be fed reasonably small meals during these first few days in hospital, which is good for you. Don't expect a roast dinner the day after your operation! Eat small amounts of good, nutritious food on a regular basis, as this will aid your recovery.

Day 6-7

If no complications have arisen, you will almost certainly be home by now. You will have worked out a way of rolling onto your side to stand up out of bed alone and will continue to progress the length of your walks round the house (even if it is by 30 seconds or so each day!). Continue with your abdominal breathing exercises and Kegel exercises at this point.

You may experience constipation, night sweats, and mood swings. These are not unique to those who have had C-sections but you need to be aware that they may occur. Walking around will make your bowels less sluggish and help you become regular again, enabling you to feel more comfortable and normal again. Additionally, walking will reduce the likelihood of developing blood clots, which can be a risk at this point.

It's also important to go to the bathroom to urinate regularly. A full bladder makes it harder for the uterus to keep contracting as it proceeds to shrink, and it can also increase pressure on the wound.

Week 2

At this point you need to base your exercise decisions on your degree of discomfort, fatigue and personal motivation. Remember that your ability to exercise is determined by the healing time of your incision and your energy levels. Over doing it, and pushing yourself too hard will lead to a longer recovery time. Begin to build up your walking and continue with the Kegel exercises, stretching and mobilizing of joints, and abdominal breathing exercises.

Weeks 3-6

This period may extend to week 8 or slightly longer depending on how quickly you have healed and how much rest you have been able to take. During this period you can start with Level 2 early progressions of abdominal exercises, and begin to increase repetitions and numbers of sets of them. Strengthening your pelvic floor and abdominal muscles are a priority after a C-section. Do not attempt sit-ups, however, and high level core exercises at this point. Just enjoy progressing slowly through the Level 2. You can also concentrate on a gentle walking program. By now you may be up to 5 to 10 minutes a day. You can progress this gradually by adding about 5 minutes a week. Doing gentle shoulder retraction exercises and chest stretches are an effective way to counterbalance the hunched-over posture many women assume when holding and feeding baby.

A few points to remember:

Make sure you keep a careful eye on your incision. The scar will be sore for a few weeks at least, but you can speed up recovery by protecting it from irritation and infection. Learn from your health visitor how to apply a light dressing to the wound, and try to wear loose tops and bottoms that don't chafe your belly. Normal sensations of itching, pulling and numbness are all to be expected so don't worry if you experience these. If you feel a lot of pain beyond what your health visitor suggests is normally expected, or if the wound gets red or oozy, you need to see a doctor immediately as these show signs of an infection.

When you're in bed, use extra pillows like you did when you were propping up your pregnant belly. You should also use extra pillows to keep you still while you sleep ensuring you don't roll over onto your incision.

Keep a pillow handy in bed and a cushion handy by the chair you usually sit in. Use this when laughing or coughing, or if you need to yawn. By pressing this against your incision and holding your abdomen, the muscles will feel much more supported and the discomfort will be reduced.

Avoid exercises that require rapid changes of direction and movements that are high impact or that are bouncy or jerky. Any injury to the area of the incision will delay the recovery process. Stick to the plan laid out here and increase the amount of walking, or the number of sets and repetitions of the core exercises if they are becoming too easy.

There may be local, specific "C-section recovery" classes that you can get involved with. It's always nice to exercise with other people who are facing the same challenges. It can be really motivating to exercise with other people who are rising to the challenge too! It can also be a chance to confidently leave the house with your baby as you know the location will be tailored for babies too. You can typically find classes at your local leisure center or, ask your health visitor for details if she knows of any in the area.

You may find DVDs that are focused on postnatal fitness that you can do at home by yourself or with one or two other friends. This can be a motivating tool and can be a way of socializing if you do this with others too.

Beyond weeks 6-8

Well done! You've successfully followed a progressive program that should have you ready to resume a higher intensity of exercise. Because you have worked hard early on and made good steady progress it will not be a shock to the system when you begin higher intensity exercise. It will simply be the next stage of progression. Progressing slowly is so important. There should never be big jumps from one level to the next, rather a flowing continuum that you move along.

You can now begin to jog, start doing activities that involve a change of direction, begin to do higher level abdominal exercises like crunches and those outlined in Level 3, and start to think about resuming sports if this is something you've enjoyed before. If not, you're perfectly placed now, to join a gym, start a new hobby or take on a new challenge. Just remember, don't jump in at the deep end, start slowly and wade through the shallow waters until you get stronger and fitter. I know that by doing this you'll gain quick improvements and see great results!

The abs myth

I just want to take this opportunity to reiterate some of the points made earlier about the abdominal muscles. During the initial period of recovery from childbirth, i.e. the first 6-8 weeks, abdominal, or more importantly core work is very important for two reasons. Firstly, your tummy has been stretched and your abs have been separated and you need to help them return to normal and recover their strength. Secondly, other than walking, there's not a whole lot you can do in the first few weeks without hurting yourself, so doing core work is a safe and sensible place to start exercising.

However, after this initial period, you do not need to keep up the same volume of isolated abdominal work. Yes, you will continue to work the core, but in a more holistic way through whole body exercises and more functional exercises.

Overworking your hip flexors, abductors, and adductors, which get worked in most 'core' exercises, can lead to over-development of these muscles. If your hip flexors are overworked, you can actually cause lower back strain because the overdeveloped hip flexors will put strain on the hip joint and pull it out of alignment.

When exercises like squats, overhead squats, lunges and many more exercises are performed with strict technique, the core is worked as a stabilizer in an isometric way. These types of exercises will not have the same negative effect of overworking the hip flexors like performing hundreds of sit-ups and crunches would. Therefore, these types of exercises are great for working your core from this point onwards.

If you are performing these types of exercises, with a few isolated abdominal exercises thrown in, and you still do not have a flat tummy, the reason is not that you have not developed the musculature. You may have a well developed core area that is stable, balanced, and strong, but has a layer of fat covering it so you do not have the flat tummy you want. If this is the case, you need to burn more fat through weight training, interval training and a good, nutritious diet not work your core more! See my chapter on food and drink to understand the importance of a clean diet that consists of unprocessed foods and keeping refined sugars to an absolute minimum.

Chapter 7 - Motivate Me!

Have you ever been really inspired by a film you've seen, an article you've read or an amazing person you know of, and decided that you're going to make some drastic changes to your life? I certainly have. You feel completely motivated, so excited you can't sleep. You want to tell everyone about your new 'thing'. It is your first thought each morning, and the last thing on your mind at night. And then, not long after, the feelings begin to fade and the busyness of life gets in the way. Before you know it, your passion has died, and you no longer think about what you were once so excited by. In time, you even forget what it was you were going to do with your life, what changes you were going to make, and why you felt so strongly about this in the first place. Don't be too hard on yourself. This is not uncommon, it often happens over and over again in life. Passions grow and fade. Life's daily challenges crowd in. Life goes on. Big changes are very hard to achieve.

I hope that you have felt really excited and motivated by the things you've read in this book. However, I have a greater hope and desire that you are able to implement them. Otherwise my efforts just get lost as information in your head, and they will never get implemented or acted upon. I am not a fan of just knowledge. Knowledge without action loses its power. My plea to you is that you read this chapter, then make a commitment, and take the first steps towards reaching your dream. Bear in mind that often, the first few steps are the hardest. Once you have established new habits and a new rhythm it makes the "right" yet difficult daily choices easier to make.

Time to make a change

One of the hurdles that we need to overcome is an aversion to change. We are afraid of change because we don't know what the exact outcome will be, and what life will look like after the change. Will you be able to cope with the change? You may fear change and try to avoid it! Alternatively, you may be a type of person that looks forward to change and revels in it. I personally like change, as I can quite easily get bored. I enjoy trying and experiencing new things and I also feel energized by change. But, no matter who we are, change can be quite difficult. Let's take a look at some points that will help us cope with change well. Let's come out smiling and not traumatized!

Taking steps towards change

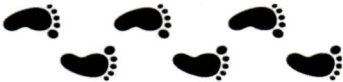

- Realize your capacity to adapt
- Honestly face your fears

- Communicate, communicate, communicate!
- Anticipate difficulties

You don't have to be a genius to work out that if the input stays the same, the output will remain the same too. You cannot expect to look and feel any different if you continue to do the same as you have always done. It's impossible. It simply will not happen. If there are no changes to your life, if you don't actually *do* something different, you will never actually achieve any change.

I encourage you to be open to change...you might be pleasantly surprised! It may not be as scary as you think.

If you are already open to change, brilliant. You have already overcome some of the barriers to losing weight and getting in shape. Personally, I think that this is a good time. Some would say that making too many changes all at once may be too difficult, but I disagree. You are already on a roll, managing multiple changes with becoming a mom. So take the opportunity, remain flexible and change other areas of your life for the better too. Once, you've got over the fact that things *are* going to be different, you will be able to cope with more change.

Find what works for you

Some people are really disciplined and motivated, and others struggle to commit to anything or to stick to their decisions. But whoever we are, we need encouragement. I believe that encouragement is one of the most powerful forces that exist. Everyone is different and therefore people will respond differently to different kinds of encouragement and motivation. Some people find things helpful that others just don't. Some people may be really impacted by one sort of encouragement, while another hardly recognizes it as encouragement. What is it that works for you? What gets your attention and resonates with you? What helps you remain true to your decisions? What helps you stay on course when it gets tough? Take a look at the following tools. I truly hope you can find what ticks your box!

Pictures & Numbers

Some individuals find images an effective form of motivation. The use of 'before and after' pictures can be a great way to compare how you looked before, with how you look now. Find a photo of yourself at a time where you were really happy with the way you looked. Hold this next to a picture of yourself that you don't like. Alternatively, compare a picture of yourself soon after giving birth, to a picture now. Look at the change in body shape and size. Use the good (or the bad) to motivate. There can be a number of stages along the way that are more subtle, but when you compare photos with dramatic differences the change is more obvious and thus more motivating.

Another good way of using images is to find a picture of how you would like to look, or find a picture of a person that you find inspirational, and place it where you will see it regularly. My husband once kept an inspirational picture of an athlete he admired in his diary. Whenever he opened it, numerous times a day, he would feel challenged and motivated by what this athlete had achieved, and it motivated him to work towards his own goals.

Seeing evidence of inches lost with a tape measure is a great way to motivate yourself and track your progress. By measuring yourself regularly, in a number of key sites on your body, you can work out the cumulative inches lost. This is a method I found particularly motivating! I have covered how best to do this in the following chapter, Making in Happen! – Monitoring your Progress. I have also talked about why weight is not always the best indicator of progress due to numerous factors, including water retention and change in body composition. Weight loss does not necessarily indicate fat loss.

Music

Music has an amazing power to affect our moods and emotions. It really can be energy giving! Athletes often listen to music to get 'in the zone' before they go out to compete, or even just to psych themselves up for a tough training session. Some may enjoy the peaceful sounds of nature, but others love running or walking listening to music. It may pump you up, or simply help pass the time, and take your mind off the hard work your body is doing. Others like to listen to quiet, calming soothing music, helping them to de-stress in order to focus and gather the energy they need to do the task in hand. Try it and see how you feel. You could formulate a playlist that works for you and name it something you find inspirational.

Quotes, Key Words & Reminders

There are numerous ways to use the power of words to motivate us. Having key words, phrases, quotes or slogans can be both encouraging and focusing. You can stick these up around the house, next to the kettle, on the bathroom mirror, above the changing table; places where you are likely to see them regularly. You may even choose to have a copy of your full exercise program stuck to your fridge!

Many people find quotes to be a powerful source of encouragement. There are thousands upon thousands of inspirational quotes out there. I have chosen a small selection for you to read. Some are focused on the early stage of having a dream, desire or vision. Others are relevant, including subjects like goal setting, making decisions, planning, preparing, stepping out, working hard, and being creative. Still others are applicable for times when you face fear, doubt, difficulty, distractions, set-backs and disappointment. Some quotes will instill hope and belief, encouraging you to keep going, to push through, and simply persevere.

These pearls of wisdom can help you grow in character, knowledge, and understanding! But most importantly quotes can help produce the results you want! Here are some, as an example, that I find helpful:

"Dreams are the seedlings of realities."
James Allen

"Aim for the moon. If you miss, you may hit a star."
W. Clement Stone

"Regardless of who you are or what you have been, you can be what you want to be."
W. Clement Stone

"Happy are those who dream dreams and are willing to pay the price to make them come true."
Anonymous

"Go confidently in the direction of your dreams. Live the life you've imagined."
Henry David Thoreau

"Dreams are renewable. No matter what our age or condition, there are still untapped possibilities within us and new beauty waiting to be born."
Dr. Dale E. Turner

"You'll never achieve your dreams if they don't become goals."
Anonymous

"If one dream should fall and break into a thousand pieces, never be afraid to pick one of those pieces up and begin again."
Flavia Weedn

"Definiteness of purpose is the starting point of all achievement."
W. Clement Stone

"You have to expect things of yourself before you can do them."
Michael Jordan

"The best time to plant a tree was 20 years ago. The second best time is now." *Chinese Proverb*

"In any moment of decision the best thing you can do is the right thing, the next best thing is the wrong thing, and the worst thing you can do is nothing."
Theodore Roosevelt

"We cannot do everything at once, but we can do something at once."
Calvin Coolidge

"Don't wait. The time will never be just right."
Napoleon Hill

"Thinking will not overcome fear but action will."
W. Clement Stone

"Systems permit ordinary people to achieve extraordinary results, predictably."
Michael Gerber

"You cannot change your destination overnight, but you can change your direction overnight."
Jim Rohn

"It always seems impossible until its done."
Nelson Mandela

"A person who aims at nothing is sure to hit it."
Anonymous

"A goal properly set is halfway reached."
Zig Ziglar

"Decisions determine destiny."
Frederick Speakman

"It's not hard to make decisions when you know what your values are."
Roy Disney

"Destiny is not a matter of chance, it is a matter of choice; it is not a thing to be waited for, it is a thing to be achieved."
William Jennings Bryan

"Stay committed to your decisions, but stay flexible in your approach."
Tom Robbins

"The only place where success comes before work is in the dictionary."
Attributed to both Vidal Sassoon and Donald Kendall

"If there is no wind, row"
Latin Proverb

"Though no one can go back and make a brand new start, anyone can start from now and make a brand new ending."
Author Unknown

"It wasn't raining when Noah built the ark."
Howard Ruff

"It is necessary; therefore, it is possible."
Giuseppe Borghese

"There is nothing in a caterpillar that tells you it's going to be a butterfly."
Buckminster Fuller

"Whether you think you can or think you can't - you are right."
Henry Ford

"There are always flowers for those who want to see them."
Henri Matisse

"Life is a challenge, meet it."
Mother Theresa

"Accept the challenges so that you can feel the exhilaration of victory."
George S. Patton

"Life's problems wouldn't be called "hurdles" if there wasn't a way to get over them."
Author Unknown

"If you want to enjoy the rainbow, be prepared to endure the storm."
Warren Wiersbe

"Never give up on yourself"
Anonymous

"When you come to the end of your rope, tie a knot and hang on."
Franklin D. Roosevelt

"You may have to fight a battle more than once to win it."
Margaret Thatcher

"Nobody trips over mountains. It is the small pebble that causes you to stumble. Pass all the pebbles in your path and you will find you have crossed the mountain."
Author Unknown

"I may not be there yet, but I'm closer than I was yesterday."
Author Unknown

"Courage is the power to let go of the familiar."
Raymond Lindquist

"Patience, persistence and perspiration make an unbeatable combination for success."
Napoleon Hill

"Success is about enjoying what you have and where you are, while pursuing achievable goals."
Bo Bennett

"Love the moment. Flowers grow out of dark moments. Therefore, each moment is vital. It affects the whole. Life is a succession of such moments and to live each, is to succeed."
Corita Kent

Even having a single word that acts as a cue for a certain mind-set or behavior is a powerful psychological tool. One of the professional skiers that my husband coaches has the word 'pleasure' written on the back of his ski gloves. This acts as a reminder to him of *why* he does what he does. It was simply the pleasure of skiing that first motivated him. He found it too easy to forget this in the heat of competition, with the pressure to achieve and his livelihood dependent on the outcome. He knows he skis best when he is relaxed and when he is doing it for the pleasure. So the key word "pleasure" is a great motivator for him and enables him to perform his best. Is there a word or phrase that would be a strong reminder/motivator for you?

Keywords to help you!

Pleasure
Confidence
Health
Fun
Life
Fit
For me and my baby
Size...(insert your dream number here that means something to you personally)
Zone in
Zone out
Calm

Having a personal mantra is a great way to remind yourself of what you're aiming for. Together with my husband Pete, we created a mantra for our boys. It is, 'Strong, Gentle, Kind'. These three words are to remind them to be the type of boys, and eventually men they are committed to being. This method can be used to remind you of the goals you are aiming for, or the values that you stand by, despite the challenges you may face.

Rewards

Knowing that there is a reward at the end of the goal can be a great motivating factor to some people who enjoy gifts and treats. If this is a tool which works for you, it is important to make sure you have mini goals along the way that you reward yourself for, as well as the reward for achieving the final goal. Ideas for these treats could include going out for a special meal, buying yourself flowers, or a new item of clothing, jewelry or any little present you like. Other ideas could include treating yourself to a spa day or a new hairstyle, a holiday ... be creative! The whole idea is to plan something that you can look forward to and make it something that you don't normally get to enjoy. Consequently it feels really special and something that you have earned. Often such rewards are extra special when other people are the ones who organize and give you the rewards (hint to all the 'significant others' who are reading this).

Imagery

This is similar to viewing an image, but instead of having a physical image this is a mental image. Here's what to do. Create an image in your mind of how you would like to look, be, live. Reflect on it, think about it, dwell on it, and maintain this in your mind's eye until it feels like it has become a reality. This method actually allows us to believe that we are really going to achieve our goal, as we've already seen the outcome in our mind before it's been realized physically. Recall the image whenever you need to know what you're aiming for and working towards, and this can help motivate you.

Positive thinking

You must remain positive towards your goal at all times. Positive thinking is a tool used by all great achievers. Ron White, the 'Memory Guy' won the USA memory championships in 2009. He accredited much of his ability and success to the fact that he listened to a Positive Affirmations CD 5 times a day, every day for 2 weeks prior to winning the USA Memory Championships. Maybe not your cup of tea! I don't know many moms who would have the time to do that. But the idea can be used. The words that others speak over you and the conversations you have with yourself are so important. In fact they are incredibly powerful. Spend time with people who are going to speak positively about your life and avoid those who do not. Protect yourself mentally and emotionally. Words can either crush your dreams or they can build your confidence and determination. The technique of positive self-talk is claimed to rewire neural pathways, which can help to eliminate your bad habits and even maximize weight loss by developing a precise focus and creating a faith in your ability to achieve what you truly desire. Experts have said that it can even overcome years of negative programming and eliminate the self-sabotaging behavior that holds people back and which brings your best efforts to a screeching halt. In essence, it re-programs the mental script that lies at the heart of many problems and difficulties, ranging from nervousness and low confidence to extreme worrying and anxiety disorders. Break the pattern of any continued negative talk and replace with positive input!

Additionally, a general positive outlook on life really helps. My husband tells me I'm a positive person, and I believe this helps me to not only achieve my goals, but to enjoy the process too. Try not focus solely on the final destination, but to enjoy the journey. Enjoy feeling fitter and stronger. Enjoy wearing the clothes you really like. Enjoy the new found confidence you feel. Enjoy the exercise. Live in the moment and enjoy life!

All these methods can be reminders or positive reinforcements that may seem 'cheesy' to some people but can be so effective as they can be tailored very personally to you. They relate to you in a deep way and cause you to recall your goal, and encourage you to persevere towards achieving the outcome that you so desire.

Bouncing back

Often when we set high targets, and fail to reach them, or fail to reach our goals as quickly as we expected to, we give up. It's important to know that hardly anyone has achieved anything without first encountering adversity or failure. If certain people had given up they would never have achieved anything of significance. All the great inventors, explorers, pioneers, and entrepreneurs overcame incredible odds so that we would be able to enjoy life as we know it now. Without them pushing on and persevering when things got tough, or trying again and again after complete failure, we would not have computers, the internet, many cures for diseases, the light bulb, the automobile, the airplane, the list goes on. We need to know how to pick ourselves up and go at it again. As Ralph Waldo Emerson said, "Our greatest glory is not in never failing, but in rising up every time we fail." I love the word *"Bouncebackability"*, coined by ex-Crystal Palace Football Club manager, Iain Dowie. Failure can be really painful and can leave us damaged and dejected. We can become bitter, or we can bounce back and become an over comer. History is full of great women and men who overcame the odds to achieve something great. Let's be people who bounce back too!

Achieving your goals will change your life. Writing this book is something I felt really passionate and excited about. I knew I wanted to help s get back in shape, offering help, motivation and advice. Writing it, however, was not always easy. If I hadn't persevered when things got tough, it would never have been finished. There were times when I lacked inspiration, when I didn't have the time, or when I felt like watching a movie or doing something else instead, but I chose to continue. I did not want this book to become an unfinished project or something that fell short of what I intended. Sometimes we just need to get on with it! Stick to your decisions as it could completely change your life.

Accountability

I believe that accountability is a great safety net against things going wrong. Without accountability we can become a Lone Ranger, doing our own thing in our own way with no regard for other people. Accountability means being inclusive and sharing our dreams and passions with one or more other people. Firstly, just one piece of advice. It's not a great idea to share your ideas with the whole world before you've achieved anything. I like to let my actions speak louder than my words, but I do share my ideas, dreams and projects with some people who I know will encourage me, and who I trust to hold me to my words.

We already know *"The mind is willing but the body is weak"* and that we will hit struggles and difficulties. Getting in shape and looking amazing may be a really big step for you. If it's a battle you're in, don't try and fight it all by yourself. Getting people to walk the journey with you will help. Is there a good friend who has also had a baby and wants to get back in shape? Follow the advice in this book together and be accountable to one another. Even if you don't know another mom, choose a close friend that you trust. You will need someone who will ask you the difficult questions, checking that you are sticking to your plan. It can be helpful to actually give them two or three specific questions to ask you every week when you meet up for a coffee. For example:

Questions to be asked

- How has your diet been this week?
- Have you stuck to your exercise plan?
- What have been the difficulties?
- How have you rewarded yourself?
- What "Me Time" have you taken?
- How can I encourage you?

By finding out what helps motivate you and keeps you on track, you are well and truly on your way to losing your baby weight and looking AMAZING!!

Chapter 8 – Make it happen! – Monitoring your Progress

We have looked in to several topics within health, happiness, fitness and weight loss after having a baby. Having highlighted key principles and offering many practical tips, I hope you will soon be enjoying your new found health and happiness which in turn, will enable you to look after yourself and your family better. It is about loving yourself, looking good and feeling great.

I do not believe in fad diets, starving yourself or 'get skinny quick' diets. I believe that following the principles laid out in this book, over time, will have a HUGE impact on your health, body and happiness. Namely, establishing healthy eating habits coupled with regular exercise and an active lifestyle will normally achieve the desired results. However, I am aware that for a few women, sadly this might not be enough. Here, therefore is Plan B.

This chapter is set out to give you the specific tools you need to actually monitor your food intake and accurately track your progress. Not everyone will need to use these specific monitoring tools, as many will gain excellent results following the earlier guidelines and advice in this book. However, I felt it necessary to provide these tools for those who do need them. It would be an injustice not to provide for those who do need close monitoring and attention to detail. For some women this may be the only way to reach the targets they desire.

If you are serious about getting in shape, and have followed the advice in my earlier chapters yet have not reached your target, this method will enable you to reach your goal. You may need to come back to re-read this chapter to ensure you follow the guidelines correctly. It is a scientific method that must be followed closely.

When using this method it is vital that you do not let it become an obsession as this can lead to developing further problems. Disordered eating and an unbalanced value on diet and fitness are not healthy and can lead to psychological stress and unhappiness. My biggest message and desire is that you are healthy and happy, therefore, please keep this in check and make sure you have a friend or group of friends who keep you accountable.

The following tools will enable you to lose weight and monitor your progress. Seeing exactly what is happening to your body as you change shape can be amazing!

The tools:

- ❖ Keeping a food Diary

- ❖ Calorie Counting

❖ Taking Body measurements

Lets learn more and unpack these tools. ...

How to keep a food diary

Decide whether you are a writer or a typer. Are you going to write things down in a notebook? Or, are going to type on a tablet, smartphone or computer? Chose which method is easiest for you and comes most naturally to you. Depending on your personality, schedule and access to gadgetry, you may prefer to keep your food journal online, in a word document or in a lovely old-fashioned notebook.

Record everything you eat it throughout the day including the calorie value of the food. If it's not practical to write everything down as you consume it, chose two moments during the day to note down what you have eaten. I would recommend one time at midday and one time in the evening. The key is that everything gets written down! As well as noting down what you eat and when, record how you feel after eating too. Did you enjoy it? Did it make you feel full? A simple way to do this would be to give a score out of 5 for enjoyment and for fullness. You may also want to record how easy or hard it was to prepare the food.

Again, please do not let this focus turn into an obsession. Showing your food diary to a friend on a regular basis will both keep you accountable for what you eat from the point of view of sticking to your plan, but it will also help avoid obsessive or compulsive behavior. If you have had an eating disorder in the past, I would not recommend you following the advice in this chapter without seeking psychological support along the way.

Here are 5 reasons why you should start keeping a food diary today:

1. Your food diary will show you what you eat

A food diary is such a great tool for anyone wanting to lose weight, but also for anyone wanting to improve their eating habits. Many women think that they know exactly what they eat each day. Some even think they could accurately guess the number of calories consumed throughout the day. But the truth is that most people eat more than three times the calories they think they have! Most of the extra calories consumed come from eating between meals. You may also be surprised at the types of food you consume or even the repetitiveness of your food choices.

2. Your food diary can help you lose weight

By seeing exactly what you eat everyday, you can begin to cut certain types of food out of your diet. You might be surprised to see that some foods that you thought were healthy actually have the highest amount of calories and do not keep you feeling full for long. By taking this into account, you can cut these calories by finding healthier alternatives for your diet. This will help you discover the foods that do keep you fuller for longer.

If you discover you are consuming numerous sugary foods as 'occasional treats', you may realize these are not actually *occasional treats* after all. Furthermore, tracking your portion size has a huge effect on calorie consumption. You may discover your portions are bigger than what you actually require. Some women eat equal amounts to their partners when that amount is not really necessary. Even when partners require significantly larger portions due to high levels of training and activity, many women unintentionally serve themselves the same amount. This can be brought to your attention when recording a food diary, when otherwise it would be left unrecognized. Additionally you may identify reasons why you eat other than for hunger, for example stress, boredom, loneliness or tiredness. Identifying these may encourage you to find other coping mechanisms.

3. Your food diary can help you plan out meals

At first, your food diary will keep track on the meals that you eat. But over time, you can actually use your food diary to plan out basic meals and snacks in order to create a more balanced and varied diet. You identify food that you really enjoy and which work for your routine. Gathering together great ideas for meals and snacks can inspire you when you do not have the time or energy to think and plan your food.

4. Your food diary will show you what you need to eat and when

You may discover you are eating very few vegetables and feel hungry a lot of the time. Because of this you may find yourself snacking regularly. You may identify that you are skipping lunch or breakfast and yet consuming more calories snacking than you would have by eating the meals. The food diary serves as a record of everything that you do, and do not eat, and *when* you eat. Identifying deficiencies in certain food groups can help you plan out your diet a little better than ever before. For example, if it becomes obvious you are consuming too little protein you can begin to change this. If you discover that you are eating high carbohydrate, high GI foods which soon leave you with low blood sugar and feeling hunger, you may change this to eat more low GI foods to maintain blood sugar levels and to avoid these sugar cravings.

5. Your food diary will keep you on track

You may not realize it right away, but over time, your food diary will actually make you want to eat healthier. Your food diary may cause you to look at food in a whole new way. Every time you write down a food that has lots of empty calories in it, you'll probably want to avoid eating it in the future. Your food diary may highlight the limited and bland diet you may presently keep and therefore encourage you to explore new foods. If you are enjoying your new, healthier diet you are more likely to adopt this food as part of your lifestyle. When something works and is enjoyable, it is sustainable!

Finally, it is important you set aside time to review your entries. A food diary doesn't help much if you never use the information! Designate a time each week to sit down and review your food journal information thoroughly. Note any trends, what you are pleased with and areas you want to change. You can also plan future meals and make new goals for the coming week.

Tricks to feeling full for longer

Satiety is that wonderfully pleasant feeling of fullness you get as you eat, when you're no longer hungry, but aren't overly stuffed or uncomfortable. You are just satisfied beyond desire. The more satisfied you feel after a meal, the less you'll eat later. The question is how to increase satiety without eating MORE?

- It's not just what you eat that can make you more satisfied—it's how you eat, too. Slow down and savor every bite. Chewing well helps digestion and gives your stomach time to signal to your brain that you have reached satiety. (This can take 20 minutes so if you wolf your food down, you can end up eating for 20 minutes past the point of being satisfied!) So take your time and enjoy every delicious bite along the way.

- Drink two glasses of water before each meal. Doing this will help fill up your stomach and thus help avoid eating more than necessary. It has been suggested that drinking water before eating can trim 60 calories off the meal.

- Include protein-rich foods at every meal. Protein is a great 'filler' so make sure you include foods such as lean meat, chicken, eggs, fish, dairy products, or beans/lentils with every meal.

- According to a study from the Department of Agricultural and Food Sciences in Zurich, Switzerland, using vinegar/vinaigrette and cinnamon for flavor (where possible) can help regulate blood sugars after meals, and help you feel full longer.

- Eat more green and orange vegetables as these contain about 90% water, filling your stomach and thus registering fullness to the brain. These vegetables, though filling, are low calorie.

- Potatoes and sweet potatoes both contain hunger-fighting resistant starch. A recent study in the British Journal of Nutrition found eating these boost satiety, helping you stay full for up to 24 hours – and eating about 320 calories less per day.

- Oats have a filling fiber compound, which helps the body release a hunger-suppressing hormone.

- Fiber-rich foods keep you feeling full for longer, therefore try swapping white carbohydrates for brown. For example, chose wholegrain cereals, whole meal bread, brown rice and whole-wheat pasta.

- Don't drink your calories. Research shows that drinks don't have the same effect on satiety as food does. For example, eat fruit rather than drinking it.

Counting Calories

Keeping a food diary where you record calories consumed really can make the difference to your weight loss success. This technique may be the key to reaching your dream.

Yes, it is possible to get a flat tummy, but this will not happen without specific help. The results rely upon following a careful method. It will happen if you follow a method and is almost impossible if you don't. If you follow a method, it's just like a formula, giving a result at the end. If you don't stick to the formula, you will not get the result you are looking for. For the majority, calorie counting is not necessary. It is time consuming and not easily sustainable long term. But, for those who feel like they have tried everything and need something more to get the results they desire, than this will work. It is a formula.

Consider mathematics formula $x + y = z$ where you are given the following instructions:

- You must produce the value $z = 5$
- You can use any positive whole number (e.g. 1,2,3,4,5,6,7,....) but no fractions or negative numbers

You therefore have a few options, you could have

$2 + 3 = 5$
or
$1 + 4 = 5$
or
$3 + 2 = 5$
or
$4 + 1 = 5$

These calculations are all correct, remain within the guidelines, and produce the desired outcome of 5. There are a few different factors that can be changed, yet give the same result. Likewise, within this method you have some flexibility, some variables you can change, but these changes must be made within the guidelines. This is a formula and there are rules. If you don't follow the rules, you will not get the desired result.

Following this method is not difficult. The problem is truly following the method, without broadening the guidelines. Those who follow their own altered method will not get the results.

If you want to lose weight, you must eat less than what your body needs for cell repair and to burn for energy. If you eat more than what your body needs, the excess food may be stored as muscle, but, mostly, it is stored as fat. Counting calories will make it easier to lose weight. If you know the calorie content of food, you can eat less high-calorie foods and more lower-calorie foods that allow you to lose weight and satisfy your nutritional requirements.

Even when calorie counting you should never be hungry. Make sure that you feel full by eating lots of low calorie foods. A general rule of thumb is "eat lots of vegetables". By doing this, you will not feel hungry and you will be taking in excellent nutrients from low calorie foods. Of course, you need to eat other foods too, but I always suggest filling up on vegetables as opposed to other food, for example bread.

So what should I do?

There is only one way of shifting unwanted areas of fat. No matter what you read elsewhere, you cannot choose an area of your body to loose fat from. Starving yourself will not get rid of the unwanted area of fat. If you do lose weight, it is likely that you will lose fat everywhere else first, leaving the fat in the unwanted area, especially round your tummy.

So here's how to loose fat...even from your tummy:

- Measure and weigh yourself (see following section on measurements)
- Calculate your basal metabolic rate (see below to calculate BMR)
- Set your daily calorie target according to your BMR, activity level, and amount of calorie deficit per day (typically 500 calories)
- Eat according to your calorie target
- Record what you eat so that you can track your progress (see section on keeping food diary above)
- Review your daily calorie target to maintain your achieved body composition
- Eat according to your new calorie target

The method of monitoring fat loss:

1. Firstly, calculate how many calories a day you are burning (see formula below).

2. You then need to keep a food diary of what you eat, aiming to eat 500 calories a day less than you need.

3. Do this for 1 week. If you are not losing weight, reduce your daily calorie intake by a further 250 calories per day. If you are losing weight, continue with the calculated deficit.

Calculating your BMR:

There are several websites where you can learn to calculate your BMR. I like this website:

http://walking.about.com/cs/calories/l/blcalcalc.htm

Enter values for height, weight and age, and your personal activity level. This will then give a value of calories you burn per day. Therefore to *maintain* weight, consume this amount of calories. To *lose* weight you should consume less than this figure to be in a state of energy deficit. To make up for this energy deficit, your body then burns the fat stored in your body.

Alternatively, you can do the calculation yourself by following these directions:

1. **Determine your height in centimeters.**
Stand with your back to a wall, with your heels touching the wall and your body straight. Have someone mark the height of the top of your head. Measure straight up to the mark from the floor with a measuring tape to find your height. If you know your height in inches, you can multiply it by 2.54 to find your height in cm.

2. **Determine your weight in kilograms.**
Use a scale that has a metric function or use a scale that measures in pounds, then convert the value in pounds to kilograms. If you know your weight in pounds, you can multiply it by .454 to find your weight in kilograms.

3. **Do the calculation**
The equation begins with a number of calories (which is set at 655 for women) that a body needs to function and then takes into account the weight, height and age of the person. As weight and height increase, so does BMR. BMR decreases with age.

Women use the following equation:

BMR = 655 + (9.6 x weight in kg) + (1.8 x height in cm) - (4.7 x age in years)

Once you know your BMR, you can multiply it by an activity multiplier to calculate your Total Daily Energy Expenditure (TDEE), which estimates the total number of calories you expend in a day. The activity multiplier for sedentary people is 1.2, lightly active people (light exercise 1 to 3 times per week) is 1.375, moderately active people (moderate exercise 3 to 5 times per week) is 1.55, very active people (hard exercise 6 to 7 times per week) is 1.725, and extremely active people (hard daily exercise or training more than once in a day) is 1.9. This will give you the total number of calories per day that you expend (on average).

BMR x Activity Multiplier = Total Daily Energy Expenditure (TDEE)

= Total number of calories burned per day

You now need to monitor and control your calorie intake by weighing your food, calculating it's calorie content and keeping your food diary. Weighing scales (for weighing food) can be purchased for about £8.

You must calculate the calorie value of your food. The calorie content for most food types can be found by typing them into one of the following websites:

http://caloriecount.about.com/

http://www.calorieking.com/

http://nutritiondata.self.com/

If you enter "egg" for example, you will be given the complete nutritional breakdown for an egg.

You must record what you consume, and not eat any more than your total daily calorie target.

As you lose weight, BMR decreases. Essentially, the lighter you are, the lower your metabolism is. It therefore becomes necessary to make adjustments to your eating plan. Alternatively, if you do not have much weight to lose, but still have body fat to lose, you can boost your BMR by increasing muscle mass through weight training. Please be aware that if you calculate that you need to cut back to less than 1200 calories a day to see weight loss, it is safer to stick to 1200 and increase your activity level. Never cut back to less than 1,200 calories per day without medical supervision. Going below your BMR can have a negative effect on both muscle retention and fat loss. Eating less than your BMR can lead to metabolic disruption. For instance, your hair, skin and nails are all 'alive' and need energy to be sustained. If you eat less than your BMR, such bodily functions become down regulated ... hence the dry skin and hair and brittle nails of many low kcal, low fat dieters. Cutting to less than 1200 calories can also lower production of important hormones (testosterone and Thyroid Stimulating Hormone), which are key to a healthy metabolism.

It is safe and realistic to aim for 500 calories a day below your TDEE. However, it is not quite as straight forward as just eating that specific number of calories. **It is important to eat the right foods and not to go hungry**. The reason many people carry more fat than is healthy for them may not be due to lack of self control, ill discipline or some character issue. Many simply act on false information. Follow the guidelines in the earlier nutrition chapter to make the best food choices.

Setting your target

If you have a lot of weight to lose you should first set a target weight and record it. Write it down and keep it somewhere safe. Once you have decided how much weight you need to lose you can aim to lose between 0.5 and 2lbs per week, but perhaps double that in the initial few weeks. The general rule of thumb is that you can lose approximately 1% of your body weight per week.

When you reach your target you must stop losing weight and eat the correct number of calories to **maintain** your new weight (this is the value initially calculated before subtracting the 500, however, I would encourage you to redo the calculation now to take into account your new weight and any changes in activity). Do not eat more, or you will **gain** weight. Do not eat less or you will continue to **lose** weight.

As you may know, you may reach your target weight but not look how you want to. You will see below that weight loss does not equal fat loss, and therefore, at some point you need to set a target for your desired measurements.

Taking Body Measurements

You will see that taking body measurements can be a better way of determining fat loss. By following the guidelines below, set a target measurement for a number of body areas, for example your waist and your hips. Be positive and decide on the size you want to be. Find out typical measurements for dress sizes (this varies depending on where you live in the world) and use these to set your goal. All women are of different heights and shapes and therefore the same measurements can look different on each individual. Therefore tailor your targets realistically with your shape! Bare in mind each dress size has a range of measurements that fit a particular size.

Following the initial stages of weight loss, I recommend taking measurements to monitor progress instead of weighing yourself. Body measurements can be a better way to track your progress and keep you motivated. You can expect to see inches lost even when the scale isn't moving. It is even possible to go down a dress size, and look slimmer, but have a slight increase in weight. This is why measuring is great, and weighing may not always reflect positive body changes. To ensure accuracy, measure in exactly the same place and under the same conditions each time. Here are some instructions and tips to help you.

Things you'll need:

- Flexible measuring tape (one from a sewing kit is perfect)
- Notebook
- Pencil

Common body measurements:

Bust: Place the measuring tape across your nipples and measure around the largest part of your chest. Be sure to keep the tape horizontal round your body.

Chest: Place the measuring tape just under your breasts/pecs and measure around the torso while keeping the tape parallel to the floor.

Waist (narrowest part): Place the measuring tape about ½ inch above your bellybutton (at the narrowest part of your waist) to measure around your torso. When measuring your waist, exhale and measure before inhaling again.

Waist (widest part): Place the measuring tape round the widest part of your waist. This is approximately where your bellybutton is.

Hips: Place the measuring tape across the widest part of your hips/buttocks and measure all the way around while keeping the tape parallel to the floor and your legs together.

Thigh: Measure around the largest part of each thigh.

Calves: Measure around the largest part of each calf.

Upper arm: Measure around the largest part of each arm (above the elbow).

Forearm: Measure around the largest part of each arm (below the elbow).

Neck: Measure around the largest part of the neck.

When taking measurements, stand tall with your muscles relaxed and your feet together.

As shown, there are many body parts you can chose to measure. I like to keep it simple, recording seven points, logging values in a little table in excel where I can calculate total inches lost:

	Week 1	Week 2	Week 3	Week 4
Bust				
Waist (narrowest part)				
Waist (widest part)				
Hips				
Forearm				
Thigh				
Calf				
Total inches				
Weight				
Inches lost since last time				
Inches lost since the start				

Initially it can be useful to measure once each week, and as the weeks pass, as inch loss slows down, I recommend measuring once every two weeks. When you have reached your target and maintenance becomes your focus, measure periodically, once a month or less. If you're happy with what you've achieved and are maintaining your new body, you do not need to continue measuring!

How to measure yourself

- When measuring, apply constant pressure to the tape (so it doesn't sag) without pinching the skin.
- Use a flexible measuring tape (plastic or cloth)
- Measure under the same conditions each time. Wearing the same clothes (pants and bra would be best), and at the same time of day
- Measure yourself in front of a mirror to make sure the tape is positioned correctly. Or, if possible, have someone else do the measuring for you.
- The exact spot from which each measurement is taken will vary slightly from person to person. To ensure accuracy, remember to take them in the same spot on your body each time.

Please remember not to get obsessed with the numbers on the scales! Losing inches means you'll be losing fat and wearing your dream size in no time! Everyone will be commenting on how great you look, and the number on the scales will suddenly seem a lot less important.

The difference between fat and weight

There are two ways that we acquire excess weight in the body. One is through the increase in muscle mass, and the other is through the accumulation of fat.

Body composition can be defined as the proportion of fat, muscle and bone that an individual's body is made up of. It can be expressed as a percentage of body fat and a percentage of lean body mass.

Body composition is important because it relates to health. Essentially, if you have obvious excess fat stored, you are less healthy. We know that two people of the same height and body weight can look completely different from each other because they have a different body composition. One may have more body fat, and the other a greater amount of muscle, yet they still weigh the same. There are some people who don't need to lose weight, but need to lose fat. A change in body composition will indicate if this fat has been lost. However, scales will not reveal this change in health. It is important to note that someone with a body composition that includes excessive body fat is more likely to suffer from weight-related health problems. Be aware that even weighing the clinically recommended weight, you can still need to lose body fat to acquire your best health.

Why is tummy fat so dangerous

Tummy fat can be an indication of the presence of visceral fat. Visceral fat is the fat that surrounds the internal organs including the gut, kidneys, liver and heart. It may not be the fat that initially motivates weight loss, but this is dangerous fat to have. As Dr. David Haslam, clinical director of the National Obesity Forum, shockingly explains: "Visceral fat may seem to be an inert lump of lard, but it's actually highly active and constantly pumping poisons into the bloodstream." Visceral fat is known to cause inflammation in the colon and the artery walls, and is a major cause of heart disease, diabetes and some types of cancer. Research even suggests that visceral fat affects mood by increasing production of the stress hormone, cortisol, and reducing levels of feel-good endorphins. So, along with potentially killing you, visceral fat, in the mean time can make you feel low!

To reduce visceral fat, it requires a reduction of total body fat. The good news is that when you diet and exercise, you can lower the amount of visceral fat much quicker than the fat on your tummy that you can pinch. Therefore, be encouraged that even when you see little change to the subcutaneous fat under the skin (which pose little health risk in comparison) you may well have decreased your visceral fat.

Why all this focus on food when I exercise regularly?

By just exercising alone, it will be impossible to lose the baby weight that you have put on, or any excess weight that you would like to get rid of. Here's why. If you go for a half an hour jog, you may burn 200 calories. One pound of fat takes 3500 calories to burn off. This is the equivalent of 17 or 18 of those 30-minute jogs, just to burn 1lb of fat!! Even if you do manage to exercise a lot, it is easy to consume more calories than you burn exercising.

This makes it sound impossible, but the truth is by combining regular exercise and good nutrition you can lose excess fat. Cutting 500 calories below your TDEE per day for one week will cause the deficit of 3500 calories i.e. 1lb fat. By combining exercise with cutting your calories, you make it possible to create a deficit without cutting all of the 500 calories through minimizing food. For example, you could cut 300 calories through food consumption (i.e. eat 300 calories less) and expend 200 calories more through exercise. This way you will create the 500 calorie deficit through a *combination* of diet *and* exercise. As you can see, losing fat will not happen in a whirlwind. You need to slowly and consistently keep chipping away. It is actually better this way. Working towards your goal slowly is sustainable both mentally and physically. Furthermore, you are more likely to sustain your new body composition in the long term.

Weight training really does help develop a healthy body composition. By lifting weights you will increase your muscles mass, which in turn impacts the amount of calories you burn when you're not doing anything i.e. increases your metabolic rate. You burn calories whilst doing the weight training, and you burn calories throughout the day as a result of the increased muscle mass!

Closing remarks

Now that you've reached the end of the book, I would suggest going back over certain sections and re-reading the information. You may want to have a pen and paper to jot down some notes or even right down your goals.

I hope that you feel inspired and excited about your new life as a mom, and not worried that your days of being sexy, slim and body confident are over. Yes, your life has changed and will never be the same again, but I believe that your best years are yet to come! I wish you all the best as you pursue your goals and live your dreams!

Miri McKnight

If you have any questions, please send me a message and I'll do my best to get back to you!

About the author

Miriam McKnight is a writer, blogger, fitness enthusiast, but most of all, a wife and busy mom of 3 boys! She did a degree in Sports Science at Loughborough University, England, and was then a Physical Education teacher for a number of years. Her life took a new direction when she had her first son, and since then, she has committed herself to helping other moms improve their quality of life through regular exercise, health and activity. She lives in Annecy, France.

Thanks

I'd like to thank everyone who has contributed to this project and who have helped me in countless ways over the months. So many people have invested their time in me and I appreciate all those who have helped me along this journey of learning through knowledge and experience. Thanks to my amazing husband, Pete for encouraging me to do this and for believing in me. Thanks to my 3 gorgeous boys for providing so much entertainment (and endless loads of dirty washing to get through!) Thanks to my parents, family and close friends for always being there for me. I love you all!

Keeping in touch

If you have enjoyed reading this book and would like to find out more about resources that I recommend, or read articles on my blog, please visit my website girlgetfit.org

I love to hear stories and testimonials of how you have felt motivated, or seen great improvements in all areas of your health and fitness. So please leave me comments on the website, or get in touch through the contact page

Printed in Great Britain
by Amazon.co.uk, Ltd.,
Marston Gate.